The 30 Day Whole Food Challenge

Essential Beginner`s Guide to Best Food, Good Health, and Easy Weight Loss;

With 100 Compliant, Simple and Delicious Recipes and 30 Day Meal Plan

AUTHOR: JESSICA TROYER

Legal & Disclaimer

The information contained in this book and its contents is not designed to replace or take the place of any form of medical or professional advice; and is not meant to replace the need for independent medical, financial, legal or other professional advice or services, as may be required. The content and information in this book have been provided for educational and entertainment purposes only.

The content and information contained in this book have been compiled from sources deemed reliable, and it is accurate to the best of the Author's knowledge, information, and belief. However, the Author cannot guarantee its accuracy and validity and cannot be held liable for any errors and omissions. Further, changes are periodically made to this book as and when needed. Where appropriate and necessary, you must consult a professional (including but not limited to your doctor, attorney, financial advisor or such other professional advisor) before using any of the suggested remedies, techniques, or information in this book.

Upon using the contents and information contained in this book, you agree to hold harmless the Author from and against any damages, costs, and expenses, including any legal fees potentially resulting from the application of any of the information provided by this book. This disclaimer applies to any loss, damages or injury caused by the use and application, whether directly or indirectly, of any advice or information presented, whether for breach of contract, tort, negligence, personal injury, criminal intent, or under any other cause of action.

You agree to accept all risks of using the information presented in this book.

You agree that by continuing to read this book, where appropriate and necessary, you shall consult a professional (including but not limited to your doctor, attorney, or financial advisor or such other advisor as needed) before using any of the suggested remedies, techniques, or information in this book.

Contents

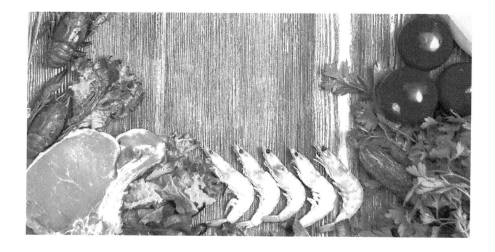

Introduction

If just open up your mind and take a peek into the world of diets that are trending these days, a certain one is known as the "Whole Food Diet" will pop up more often than not.

While the name of other diets such as Alkaline, Ketogenic or even Paleo diets, somewhat makes sense, the words "Whole Food Diet" usually tend to fill up the head of an unknown individual with nothing but confusion!

However, soon after doing a little bit of research, things start to become pretty clear, and individuals who are interested in finding their next "Groundbreaking" and "Revolutionary" diet soon realize that the Whole Food diet is hands down, the healthiest and most effective diet to date!

If you are an individual who has been searching for a book that offers the perfect blend of accessibility and technical information, then it's safe to say that you have arrived at the right place!

Let me first thank you for purchasing this book. Your small gesture of kindness will go a long way in supporting me in my future endeavors.

I have tried to design this book in such a way that, it can seamless entertain readers of every level. Regardless whether you are an amateur in the field of Whole Food diet or an expert, you are bound to find something useful here.

The whole book has been broken down into three parts, and each part is made up of individual bite-sized chapters.

The first part of the book deals with the whole concept of the Whole Food diet and will try to explain the fundamental rules and regulations of the diet.

A very nifty sample meal plan will be included in second part that will help you to understand just how you should design your future meal plans to maximize its effectiveness. The meal plans will also give you an idea of how you create your weekly shopping lists as well.

And to top everything off, the last part will focus on the collection of absolutely delicious and mouthwatering recipes!

All of the recipes used in the meal plan can be found in the recipe galore of this book. So, you won't have to go recipe hunting on the web either!

I welcome you to the world of Whole Food Diet!

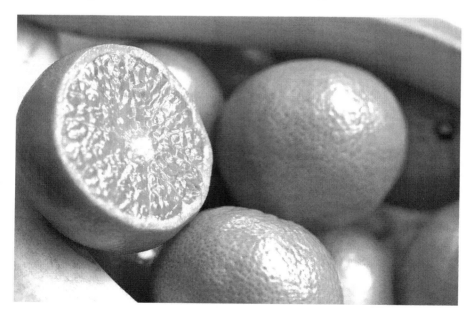

Part 1: The Fundamentals of Whole Food Diet

As mentioned in the introduction, the first part of this book is all about making yourself comfortable by helping you to wrap the concept of the Whole Food Diet around your head.

Throughout this part, you will find information that will cover topics such as:

- The basic definition of the Whole Food Diet
- Get to know the different food groups and the standards of food that you should try to pursue
- Understand the food groups that make you unhealthier
- Understand the restrictions of the diet and get to know the food groups that you are allowed to eat and the ones that you are required to get rid of.
- Understand how you should deal with the Whole Food Diet if you are breastfeeding or pregnant
- Get to know what you should do after your 30-day Whole Food challenge is complete
- Learn how to prepare your kitchen by having the most crucial components for a better experience
- Know about some side effects, which you should be aware of
- Get some tips on how you can successfully carry out your Whole Food journey
- Know about the advantages of following a Whole Food Diet

Chapter 1: What Exactly is Whole Food Diet?

Considering the recent statistics, more than 10,000 people all around the world have already jumped into the Whole Food Diet bandwagon and are already sharing their "Life Changing" experiences.

So, naturally, the first question that pops in mind is obviously the most basic one.

"What exactly is a Whole Food diet?"

Whole Food diet is a month-long (30 days) program that encourages an individual to get rid of a number of specific food groups in order to purify or "Cleanse" the whole ecosystem of the body.

This particular diet promises to bless an individual with a large array of benefits that are both physical and psychological.

This systemic reset will seamlessly allow your body to re-invigorate the metabolic, digestive and defensive mechanism of the body and in turn, make the whole body much healthier in the long run.

The 30 Day Whole Food Challenge program tries to fully "RESET" the whole metabolic system of the body and completely reshape how you interact with your food on a daily basis.

Generally speaking, the menu of a Whole Food diet very closely resembles that of a Paleo Diet, which promotes a high protein and low carb diet.

But the Whole Food Diet is much more advanced and strict in terms of elimination. Unlike Paleo, there's no option to cheat here. For one whole month, you are required to get rid of your indulgences.

Food groups such as inflammatory groups such as grains, dairy, sugar, alcohols, and legumes are required to be completely eliminated.

Not to mention, junk foods such as Burgers or even Pizza are off the table as well.

The restrictions of the diet should not be regarded as a limiting factor to your lifestyle, but rather a means through which you will be able to re-orient your food habits so that you can enjoy cleaner and simpler foods.

As much difficult as the whole journey may sound like, I will try my very best to provide you with the guidelines required to make your journey as smooth as possible.

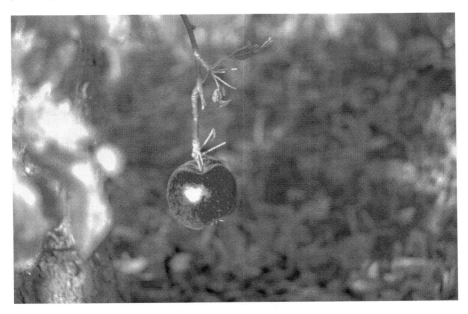

Chapter 2: Why Should You Follow a Whole Food Diet?

You must be wondering now, why should you follow a Whole Food diet right? I mean, in the first chapter I have already talked a bit about how thousands of people are already in the Whole Food cycle, but I didn't really talk about the benefits, right?

While the list of benefits that can be achieved through a proper Whole Food reset would easily fill up even the largest bucket, I am going to list out some of the more prominent ones here that are bound to encourage you for a better future.

Improved skin, nails and hair condition: Let's start with one of the most unexpected benefits first! Once you start to cut down the unhealthy foods from your body, the condition of your skin and nails will greatly start to improve.

More available energy to spend: It has been seen that people who are on a Whole Food diet tend to have about 3 times more energy than a person who isn't. This is primarily because you are fueling up your body with a 100% pure green energy.

However, it should be noted that the energy won't necessarily be instantaneous. You will feel a little bit of sluggishness during the first week or so, but once your body adjusts itself to the changed diet, you soon feel the surge of energy flowing through your veins.

Will help you to trim down excess weight: Since you are completely getting rid of sugar alongside any sort of junk foods! The Whole Food Diet will have a huge impact in the long run when it comes to trimming down your fat. Through Whole Food Diet, you are essentially promoting your mind to pay more attention to the food that you are eating, thus eliminating more fatty foods from your list, which will, in turn, cause your body to eventually lose weight and attain the physique that you have been dreaming of! If you just do a little research, you are bound to find thousands of stories of man and women successfully losing their weight through Whole Food diet.

It will improve your sleeping condition: The Whole Food Diet actually goes a long way when it comes to improving and regulating the hormones in your body. This will help you to improve how your body manages its internal sleep timer and generally improve your sleeping patterns.

It will help you to stay focused all day: When you are gathering your food from quality resources, it will keep pumping you up with energy at a slow, yet steady rate. This will keep you healthy and energized all throughout the day.

The diet will fully break any sentimental attachment you may have with food: Emotions tend to control the type of food that you swallow more often than you might think. If you are feeling sad, then you will soon go for a chocolate milkshake! If you are happy, then you might go for something more invigorating like a pancake donut!

The Whole Food Diet will help you to make more logical decisions and help you to control your food intake.

It will make you more sexually active and fertile: Too much sugar causes lots of problems, including body inflammation.

Since a Whole Food diet will greatly reduce the sugar intake, it will help you to lower down the symptoms of diseases such as endometriosis (a disease that affects female sex organs).

This, in turn, will improve your fertility and make you feel more sexually active.

It will help you to tackle Anxiety and Depression: Depression is a very common problem these days, and a more balanced link between your brain and food intake will improve the condition.

It will help you to reverse serious disease symptoms: Multiple diseases such as diabetes, cerebral palsy or even multiple sclerosis can be dealt with while being on a Whole Food diet. Patients with such diseases have shown great improvement from these chronic diseases while on a Whole Food diet.

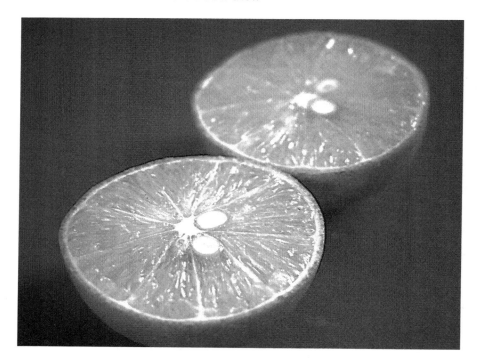

Chapter 3: Understanding Your Food

As mentioned earlier, the success of your 30 Day Whole Food Challenge will largely depend on how well you are able to eliminate the unhealthy food from your life.

The ingredients and recipes that are chosen for the Whole Food Diet strictly rely on four principles that assess the standard of the food that you are eating.

In short, foods that satisfy these four principles are the good ones! (the list will be provided soon):

- The food should promote a healthy psychological response from your body
- The food should promote a healthy hormonal response
- The food should improve the quality of your gut
- The food should improve your immune function and minimize your inflammation

Based on those standards, the food groups that you are allowed to use on the 30 Day Whole Food Challenge include:

Vegetables: Don't compromise on vegetables! Including potatoes as well! There's no restriction here.

Fruits: It should be noted that fruits are allowed in moderation in a Whole Food diet as they are sugar machines.

Unprocessed Meats: Always go for unprocessed meats as processed foods tend to add sugar and other preservatives. However, Sausage works.

Seafood: Fish and Shellfish are allowed on a Whole Food diet.

Eggs: Eggs should be on your breakfast list as well.

Nuts and Seeds: All nuts are fully allowed during your 30 Day Whole Food Challenge except peanuts (as they are legumes).

Oil and Ghee: You can go for unprocessed extra virgin olive oil and unprocessed extra virgin coconut oil and Ghee.

Coffee: This should come as a great joy to coffee lovers! While you are on the 30 Day Whole Food Challenge, you are allowed to go for coffee. Just make sure you don't add any milk products or sugar. You may use almond milk though.

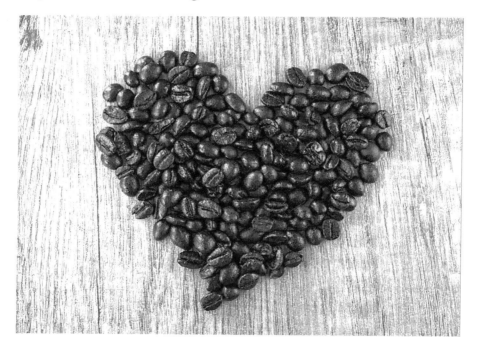

That being said, the following food groups are completely restricted:

Dairy: This means that you are not allowed to go for cow milk, cheese, cream, yogurt, sour cream, butter or even kefir. Only ghee is an exception.

Grains: Such as corns, rice, wheat, quinoa, millet, amaranth, sorghum, buckwheat, sprouted grains and Bulgur are off the table.

Alcohol: This might come as a little bit harsh, but alcohol is completely restricted during 30 Day Whole Food Challenge, either for drinking or cooking.

Legumes: Legumes such as soy sauce, tofu, peanuts, and lentils are off the table as well.

Extra Sugar: Any added sugars (even artificial sweeteners) are to be avoided. Honey, agave, maple syrup, Stevia are all off the table.

Carrageenan, Sulfites or MSG: Try to avoid processed foods.

Any kind of "Junk" Food: Junk and baked foods are strictly prohibited during a 30 Day Whole Food Challenge, even if they are made using Whole Food Diet compliant ingredients.

As an exception though, you can have:

- Fruit juice
- Green beans, sugar snap peas, and snow peas
- Vinegar

The Whole Food Diet is completely designed around all of these food groups in order to target and improve specific parts of our health.

To break them down, these include:

Breaking an unhealthy relationship with food: The Whole Food Diet will help you clear up any psychological or emotional relation that you might have with unhealthy food. By eliminating nutrient, poor, calorie dense food that promotes overconsumption.

Improve metabolism: The meal plan and regulation that are offered by the Whole Food Diet will greatly help you to restore your

19

hormonal levels and regulate the blood sugar. Over time, this will help your body to use fat as a fuel. As a result, your energy levels will increase, and you will trim a bit of fat in the process as well.

Improve digestive system: The gut will be greatly helped by your Whole Food program as foods that often tend to prevent the gut from working properly are completely eliminated from the diet. This gives your gut time to heal and calm down your immune system in the process.

Soothe and calm an over-reactive Immune System: The Whole Food Diet is really an Anti-Inflammatory diet that helps to calm down an over-reactive immune system. Various symptoms such as aches and pains are greatly relieved during this diet.

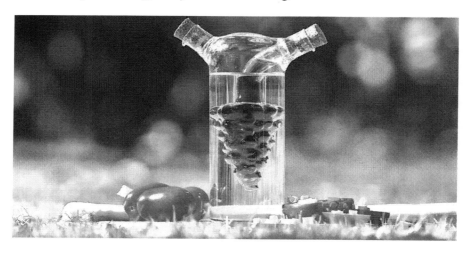

Chapter 4: General Whole Food Diet Guidelines for Breastfeeding and Nursing Mother

While you are nursing or are pregnant, it is of paramount importance you maintain a good flow of food to ensure that your body is getting enough nutrition for the growing baby.

Diets that are healthiest for you does not necessarily mean that it's going to be the best for your baby.

And Whole Food diet does not really fall on the good spectrum when it comes to your baby.

So, certain changes are to be made to your Whole Food diet in order to make it better suitable for your baby and you.

While Pregnant

When it comes to pregnancy though, the Whole Food Diet doesn't really need a whole lot of modification; however, it is essential that some minute adjustments are made to the diet.

It should be noted that a high-protein diet such as a Whole Food, isn't really that healthy for the growing baby. Generally speaking, pregnant women should have a stricter control over protein intake, and it should not exceed about 20% of the total consumed calorie.

Key steps that you should keep in mind:

- As mentioned earlier, make sure to create a diet plan that is low in protein
- Just in case if you lean more towards a higher protein diet, you should try to eat more fat and carbs to make for missing calories

- After the first 3 months of your pregnancy, try to add an extra 300 calories to your diet in order to make sure that your baby is properly fed
- While usually, Whole Food Diet has a strict policy against snacking, pregnancy will require you to resort to smaller meals throughout the day in order to keep everything in check
- Mercury-containing food (such as Tuna, Marlin, Raw Eggs, Swordfish and/or raw meat) is to be avoided

Some tips to avoid morning sickness:

- Try to keep most or all of your required groceries at home. It will prevent you from needing to go to the shopping market every day and will give you more time to breathe and relax.
- Try to be more flexible when it comes to managing your meal plan. During pregnancy, you will need to alter your meal plan as required.
- Make sure to follow your instinct. If you think that the Whole Food Diet is leaving you exhausted or underfed, then don't hesitate to take a break and go on a regular diet to keep yourself and the baby packed.

Some supplements to consider:

Before taking any supplements, make sure to discuss the diet thoroughly with your dietician:

- Make sure to go for prenatal vitamins to get the appropriate levels of vitamins and minerals
- Try to go for supplementing yourself with about 300mg of DHA per day
- Go for COD Liver Oil as they are excellent source of Omega -3 fats and Vitamins such as A, D, and K2
- Vitamin D3 plays a great role when it comes to keeping you healthy during pregnancy
- If possible, then go for some healthy homemade bone broth as they are great source of calcium, magnesium, phosphorus

- Vitamin B Complex will maintain a healthy growth of your baby
- Liver pills are excellent sources of Vitamins like A, D and E alongside choline and Iron

While Breastfeeding

Unlike pregnancy, a Whole Food diet is excellent for nursing mothers. The diet will help you to stay healthy and energetic while keeping your immune system in tip-top shape.

Your baby will be able to get all the required micronutrients as well.

Some tips to maintain a nutritious breast milk supply for your baby:

- Make sure to keep your breast empty. Meaning try to feed your baby according to his/her desire and/or empty your breast using a pump after you feed your baby. An empty breast will result in faster milk generation.
- While breastfeeding, make sure to keep your daily calories intake above 1800, otherwise, it might result in less milk production.
- Keep your daily carb above 100g
- Make sure to keep drinking as much water as you can
- Just like pregnancy, you should try to take small sized meals throughout the day. Make sure to include a good amount protein, fat and carbs in your diet as well. The limitation of protein is only needed during pregnancy.

Supplements to consider while breastfeeding

- Go for COD Liver Oil as they are excellent source of Omega -3 fats and Vitamins such as A, D, and K2
- Vitamin D3 plays a great role when it comes to keeping you healthy during pregnancy
- If possible, then go for some healthy homemade bone broth as they are great source of calcium, magnesium, phosphorus

Chapter 5: Preparing Your Kitchen for the Journey

Before diving into the recipes, it is essential that you know about the utensils that you are going to need in order to properly prepare the meals ahead.

I am pretty sure that you already have the following items in your kitchen, but if you are a complete beginner! Then this brief chapter will help you out a lot.

Don't stress too much though! Just relax and try to keep things handy.

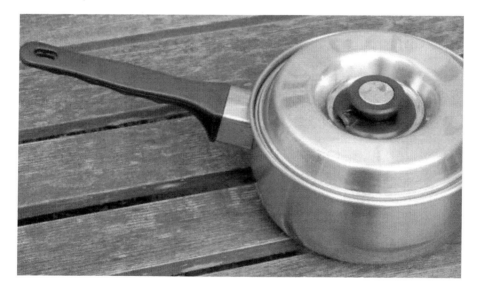

Saucepan: 1-2 quarts of small saucepan

Dutch oven: 3-4 quart Dutch oven for large dishes

Frying Pans: Frying pans (skillets)

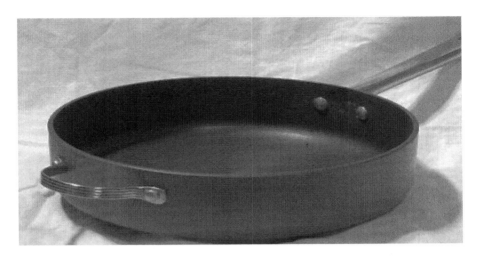

Saute Pan: High-walled Saute pans should be on your list as well.

Strainer: Strainer for allowing you to drain water from boiled vegetables or broth, which can also be used as a steamer rack with large sized stock pot

Measuring cups and spoons: A set of measuring cups and spoons, keep larger sized glass measuring cup as well

Baking Sheet: Baking sheets that will be required for roasting vegetables or meat

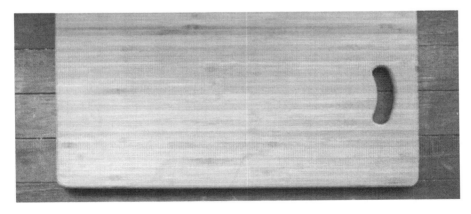

Cutting Board: A nice cutting board as you will be doing a lot of chopping. If possible, a wooden or bamboo surfaced one as they leave less bacterial residue

Knives: Try to go for some high-quality knives. A paring knife, an 8-inch chef's knife, and a long slicing knife should be on the top of your list.

Food Processor: A food processor might sound like an expensive tool, but you will find some good fits within your budget. You should keep one handy as they will very easily help you to chop up or shred ingredients to a fine consistency.

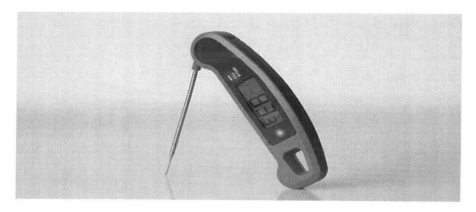

Meat Thermometer: A good quality meat thermometer to make sure that your meat and poultry are cooked to the right degree.

Parchment Paper: Parchment paper for lining up your baking sheets and dishes. This is much better than aluminum foil as it keeps your dishes cleaner

Garlic Press: Mincing garlic might just become one of your most hated tasks during your culinary adventures. A Garlic Press will help you to mince your garlic in seconds.

Julienne Peeler: This will help you create amazing vegetable noodles that will greatly add a hefty dose of variety to your Julienne Peeler.

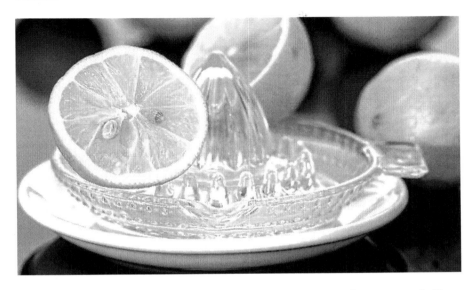

Citrus Juicer: This will help you to squeeze lemon and lime seamlessly.

Zester: Some recipes in this book might call require you to use zest. A zester will easily create tiny pieces orange or lemon peels for your meal.

Meat Tenderizer: This is a very handy and inexpensive kitchen tool that looks like a hammer. It will help you to flatten your meat using one end and texturize them using the other.

Chapter 6: After the 30 Days

So, you are done with your Whole Food challenge right? Imagining what you should do now?

Well, fear not!

According to the guidelines of a Whole Food diet, there are actually 3 more steps that you should keep in consideration to the fully enjoy the benefits of a Whole Food diet. In this chapter, we will be talking about the different steps individually.

Let's start off with the 2nd step first.

Step 2: The Step of Reintroduction

The second step, simply known as "Reintroduction" is a very crucial part of a Whole Food journey.

Once you are done with step 1 (The Whole Food Challenge), the next step is to simply make up a meal plan for the next 10 days, where you are going to re-introduce some of the food that you have been avoiding for the past month.

Throughout this gradual introduction, you will get the chance to properly assess how these foods are now reacting to your metabolic levels and evaluate, which ones are going to help you maintain a healthy body in the long run.

The plan of re-introduction will usually require you to re-introduce 1 food group at a time, to ensure that you are still heavily relying on your Whole Food diet.

You can think of this stage as somewhat of a scientific trial that you are running in order to check if any of those previously canceled food group are worth bringing back.

This means that you are not to combine multiple major food groups together. For example, you can have a slice of toasted bread with peanut butter! Rather, you should either go for bread or peanut butter.

Regardless of what you do, pay very close attention to how your body reacts and be the best judge of yourself.

A sample schedule for 10 days might include:

Day 1: You may start off by trying to re-introduce legumes and evaluate how they work.

Day 4: After a 3 days trial run, select the legumes that you want to keep and move on to re-introducing Non-Gluten grains such as corn tortilla chips or white rice.

Day 7: This should be followed by an evaluation of Dairy products. Some cheese or ice creams are to be considered during this phase.

Day 10: Finally, you should evaluate Gluten-Containing Grains to see how they react to your body.

It should be noted that throughout all of these process, you are to stick to your usual Whole Food diet while only including the experimental food group that is being assessed.

Step 3: Sharing is Caring

The Whole Food Diet has a very robust community of inspiring individuals whose lives were completely changed through a Whole Food diet.

Once you are done tallying and recording the amazing changes that have occurred in your life, the best step to do next is to share your story with other Whole Food Diet members who might be going through a similar situation such as yours.

You might be pleasantly surprised to see just how much of an impact your story might make in the life of someone else.

Regardless of the fact that your story is big or small, dramatic or simple! Just share it with your local Whole Food Diet community or online.

Even if a single person reads it and says "Hey, he/she is just like me!"

Then you will feel proud that your story has touched another human being.

A good tip to make your story even more powerful is to add a picture that might show your amazing transformation.

Some pointers that you may include in your story may include:

- How you brought control over your food eating habits
- How Whole Food Diet helped to eliminate various symptoms or conditions
- How the biomarkers such as triglycerides, blood pressure or blood sugar level improved
- How the Whole Food Diet helped you to trim down your weight and gain back your confidence
- How Whole Food diet helped you to be at peace with yourself
- How you were able to transfer the Whole Food Diet habits to other aspects of your life and so on…

The ideas are boundless! The only limiting factor here is your will to share your experience with the world.

Step 4: The journey afterward

You should always take the 30-day Whole Food journey as a starting point for something great in your life. This diet won't help you to completely eradicate the damage that has already been done to your body by past food decision.

However, it can surely help you to rectify your mistakes and ensure that your body stays in tip-top shape in the coming days.

But let's face it, we are human beings, and at some point, we are bound to lose ourselves to the temptation of savory and delightful meals right?

What should you do then? It is not always possible to stick to a plan like a robot!

Therefore, a good strategy moving forward should include the following steps:

- Keep focusing on your Whole Food based meals every single day as long as you can without breaks or any kind of "Cheat Day." Should the lust for sugar come creeping back to you, go for something very minute, just enough to control the temptation. But don't give it!
- However, should you stumble upon something that is just too irresistible or perhaps something that is culturally or religiously important to you, make a small exception and assess if the food is actually worth it? If it helps, then you can follow the below given that it will greatly help you assess the food and decide if eating it would be a good idea.
- In the case where you have decided to indulge the meal, take your time to savor it. Eat consciously without ruining your diet. A good way is to eat just as much as you need to ensure that you are not feeling uncomfortable anymore and keep the rest for later use.
- Once you are done with your meal, don't feel guilt or shame! These things happen. Tell yourself that you have made a conscious decision and given yourself some slack. Moving forward, try to bring more control and stick to your Whole Food diet as much as you can.

Word to the wise

Sometimes in your life, you might come across various occasions where eating savory food is unavoidable. Maybe during a vacation or even during a stressful time!

An easy way to get back from such sudden "Dirty" food eating sessions is to simply go on a shorter diet with a very strict Whole Food compliant meal to get your body back on the track.

You may go on a 14-day Whole Food or even 7-day Whole Food diet, whichever helps you to remove the feeling of guilt and make you feel awesome again!

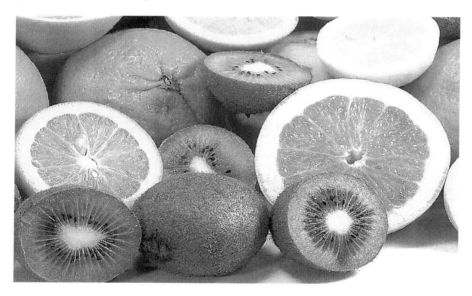

Chapter 7: Some Tips and Side Effect You Should Know About!

With all of that out of the way, here are some bonus tips for you to ensure that you can fully enjoy your Whole Food diet as efficiently as possible!

- Always make sure to read the labels before you eat anything to ensure that you are not eating anything that is not Whole Food Diet compliant
- Try to plan your meals for the next few days as early as possible. It will help you to stay less stressed and make life easier for you
- Try to share your experience and your Whole Food journey with as many friends and family members as you can. You may not realize it now, but a little support from loved ones will go a long way
- Don't replace junk foods with Whole Food Diet compliant junk foods! Make sure to completely eliminate any kind of junk food (Whole Food Diet compliant or not)
- Make sure to go for Carbs, Healthy Fats and Protein at every meal
- Try to avoid measuring your weight during the 30 days. Instead, focus on keeping your body healthy rather than the change in weight

Some side effects to know about

If you have already experimented or even explored through a number of different diets, then you are sure to know that every diet is accompanied by at least a minute number of side effects.

Naturally, this might make you wonder if the Whole Food diet has any side effects as well.

The good news here is that the Whole Food diet does not necessarily pose any serious threat to the body! However, there have been reports of some very minor symptoms that are experienced by newcomers.

Below, I will list them so that you may rest comfortably, knowing that they will soon pass away.

These symptoms usually show up within the first 14 days of the diet and soon go away once the body habituates itself to the new diet:

- Minor headaches
- Feeling of lethargy
- Sleepiness
- General Crankiness
- Brain Fog
- Food Cravings
- Minor Breakouts
- Minor Bloating

With all of those out of the way, here are some tips which you should keep in mind in order to make your Whole Food journey as pleasant as possible.

Part 2: A Generalized Meal Plan

With all that information, you must really be excited to jump into the recipes and start your journey right?

Well, the following Meal Plan will help you to mentally prepare yourself for the upcoming 30 days and plan what meal you are going to eat. Keep in mind that all of the recipes found in the meal plan are taken from the book.

You can easily alter the recipes according to your preferences and create your own meal!

After each meal, I have included a short list of the required ingredients for the recipes, which will help you to shop for the meals ahead of time!

Bon Appetite!

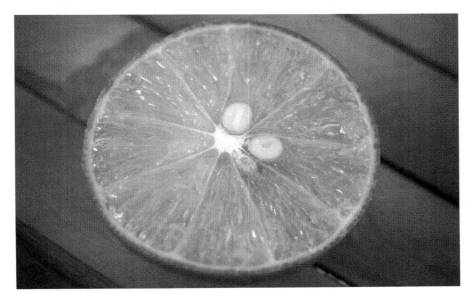

Chapter 8: The Epic Meal Plan

Week 1 Meal Plan

Week 1	Breakfast	Lunch	Dinner
Day 1	Black Berry And Coconut Chia Pudding	Law Breaking Simple Asparagus	Supremely Fascinating Lemon Chicken
Day 2	Feisty Grilled Artichokes of America	Surprisingly Healthy Broccoli Soup	Feisty Crispy Fish Fillets
Day 3	Sautéed Zucchini for a Refreshing Morning	Uncle Adam's Turkey and Vegetable	Mustard Drizzled Chicken
Day 4	Feisty Grilled Artichokes of America	Surprisingly Healthy Broccoli Soup	Mustard Drizzled Chicken
Day 5	Black Berry and Coconut Chia Pudding	Law Breaking Simple Asparagus	Feisty Crispy Fish Fillets
Day 6	Feisty Grilled Artichokes of America	Surprisingly Healthy Broccoli Soup	Supremely Fascinating Lemon Chicken
Day 7	Sautéed Zucchini for a Refreshing Morning	Uncle Adam's Turkey and Vegetable	Mustard Drizzled Chicken

Reference for Week 1 Shopping List

For Breakfast

Recipe 1: Black Berry and Coconut Chia Pudding

- ½ a cup of blackberries
- 3 tablespoons of chia seeds
- 1 cup of unsweetened almond milk
- ¼ teaspoon of 100% pure vanilla powder
- 1 tablespoon of unsweetened shredded coconut

Recipe 2: Sautéed Zucchini for a Refreshing Morning

- 1 tablespoon of extra virgin olive oil
- ½ of a diced red onion
- Salt as needed
- Pepper as needed
- 4 halved and sliced Zucchini
- ½ a pound of fresh sliced mushrooms
- 1 diced tomato
- 1 minced clove of garlic
- 1 teaspoon of Italian seasoning

Recipe 3: Feisty Grilled Artichokes of America

- 2 large sized artichokes
- 1 quartered lemon
- ¾ cup of extra virgin olive oil
- 4 chopped up garlic cloves
- 1 teaspoon of salt
- ½ a teaspoon of ground black pepper

For Lunch

Recipe 1: Law Breaking Simple Asparagus

- 1 pound of trimmed asparagus
- 1 tablespoon of extra virgin olive oil
- Salt as needed

- Pepper as needed

Recipe 2: Surprisingly Healthy Broccoli Soup

- 1 tablespoon of extra virgin olive oil
- 1 chopped up large onion
- 3 peeled and chopped garlic
- 10 ounce of frozen broccoli
- 1 peeled and chopped potato
- 4 cups of chicken broth
- ¼ teaspoon of ground nutmeg
- Salt as needed
- Pepper as needed

Recipe 3: Uncle Adam's Turkey Vegetables!

- 4 green bell pepper with tops removed and deseeded
- 1 pound of ground turkey
- 2 tablespoons of extra virgin olive oil
- 1/2 of a chopped onion
- 1 cup of sliced mushroom
- 1 chopped up zucchini
- ½ of a red chopped bell pepper
- ½ of a yellow chopped bell pepper
- 1 cup of fresh spinach
- 14 ounce of drained tomatoes
- 1 tablespoon of tomato paste
- Italian seasoning
- Garlic as needed
- Salt as needed
- Pepper as needed

For Dinner

Recipe 1: Supremely Fascinating Lemon Chicken

- 2 skinless and boneless chicken breast halves cut up into 2-inch pieces
- ¼ piece of juiced lime

- ½ a lemon juiced
- 4 tablespoons of Dijon mustard
- Freshly ground black pepper
- Creole-style seasoning

Recipe 2: Feisty Crispy Fish Fillets

- 1 whole egg
- 2 tablespoons of prepared yellow mustard
- 1/2 a teaspoon of salt
- 1 and a ½ cup of instant mashed potato flakes
- ¼ cup of extra virgin olive oil
- 6 ounce of fillets

Recipe 3: Mustard Drizzled Chicken

- 4 pieces of skinless and boneless chicken breast
- 1 cup of prepared mustard
- 6 ounce of French Fried onions

Week 2 Meal Plan

Week 2	Breakfast	Lunch	Dinner
Day 1	Surprisingly Cool Omelet Muffins	The Old Folk's Aloo Phujia	Fire and Ice Watermelon Salsa
Day 2	Suspenseful BLT Egg Salad	Golden Rose Summer's "Beach Party Special" Shrimp	The Best Trustworthy Brussels Sprouts
Day 3	Authentic Whole Food Compliant Baked Egg	Healthy Bunch of Garlic, Onion, Cabbage and Rhyming Bacon	Catchy Brazilian Fish Stew
Day 4	Authentic Whole Food Compliant Baked Egg	The Old' Folk's Aloo Phujia	Fire and Ice Watermelon Salsa
Day 5	Suspenseful BLT Egg Salad	Golden Rose Summer's "Beach Party Special" Shrimp	The Best Trustworthy Brussels Sprouts
Day 6	Surprisingly Cool Omelet Muffins	Healthy Bunch of Garlic, Onion, Cabbage and Rhyming Bacon	Catchy Brazilian Fish Stew
Day 7	Authentic Whole Food Compliant Baked Egg	The Old Folk's Aloo Phujia	Fire and Ice Watermelon Salsa

Reference for Week 2 Shopping List

For Breakfast

Recipe 1: Surprisingly Cool Omelet Muffins

- 8 pieces of eggs
- 8 ounce of crumbled cooked ham
- 1 cup of diced red bell pepper
- 1 cup of diced onion
- ¼ teaspoon of salt
- 1/8 teaspoon of ground black pepper
- 2 tablespoons of water

Recipe 2: Suspenseful BLT Egg Salad

- 1 piece of avocado
- 6 pieces of hardboiled egg
- ¾ cup of grape tomatoes cut up into halves
- 4 strips of bacon cooked crispy
- ½ a cup of chopped green onion
- 2 teaspoons of garlic powder
- ½ a teaspoon of sea salt

Recipe 3: Authentic Whole Food Compliant Baked Egg

- 1 cup of water
- 1 cup of marinara sauce
- 4 pieces of eggs

For Lunch

Recipe 1: The Old Folk's Aloo Phujia

- 1 chopped up onion
- ¼ cup of vegetable oil
- 1 pound of cubed and peeled potatoes
- 1 teaspoon of salt
- ½ a teaspoon of cayenne pepper
- ½ teaspoon of cayenne pepper
- ½ teaspoon of ground turmeric
- ¼ teaspoon of ground cumin
- 2 chopped up tomatoes

Recipe 2: Golden Rose Summer's "Beach Party Special" Shrimp

- 1/3 cup of extra virgin olive oil
- 3 sliced garlic cloves
- 1 teaspoon of red pepper flakes
- 2 teaspoons of paprika
- 2 pound of deveined (shell-on) jumbo shrimp
- ¼ cup of lemon juice
- 2 tablespoons of chopped fresh basil
- ½ a teaspoon of salt
- ¼ teaspoon of black pepper

Recipe 3: Healthy Bunch of Garlic, Onion, Cabbage And Rhyming Bacon

- 6 large sized chopped bacon
- 1 diced large onion
- 2 minced garlic cloves
- 1 large cabbage head sliced and cored
- 1 tablespoon of salt
- 1 teaspoon of ground black pepper
- ½ a teaspoon of onion powder
- ½ a teaspoon of garlic powder
- 1/8 teaspoon of paprika

For Dinner

Recipe 1: Fire and Ice Watermelon Salsa

- 3 cups of chopped up watermelon
- ½ a cup of chopped up green bell pepper
- 2 tablespoons of lime juice
- 2 tablespoons of chopped up fresh cilantro
- 1 tablespoons of chopped up jalapeno pepper
- ½ a teaspoons of garlic salt

Recipe 2: The Best Trustworthy Brussels Sprouts

- 1 and a ½ pound of Brussels sprouts with ends trimmed up

- 3 tablespoons of extra virgin olive oil
- 1 teaspoon of kosher salt
- ½ a teaspoon of finely ground black pepper

Recipe 3: Catchy Brazilian Fish Stew

- 3 tablespoons of lime juice
- 1 tablespoon of ground cumin
- 1 tablespoon of paprika
- 2 teaspoons of minced garlic
- 1 teaspoon of salt
- 1 teaspoon of black pepper
- 1 and a ½ pound of tilapia fillet cut up into chunks
- 2 tablespoons of extra virgin olive oil
- 2 chopped onions
- 4 sliced large bell peppers
- 16 ounce of diced and drained tomatoes
- 16 ounce of coconut milk
- 1 bunch of chopped off cilantro

Week 3 Meal Plan

Week 3	Breakfast	Lunch	Dinner
Day 1	A Bowl of Zucchini Zoodles	Ever so Popular Collard Greens	Craziest Tom Ka Gai Ever!
Day 2	Squash Salad for Green Lovers	Very Tangy Avocado Cucumber Salad	Steamed Cod Fish With Bizarre Lemon
Day 3	Fancy Broccoli Roasts	Obligatory Yellow Squash Of Magic	Spicy Harissa Infused Magnificent Chicken
Day 4	A Bowl of Zucchini Zoodles	Ever so Popular Collard Greens	Craziest Tom Ka Gai Ever!
Day 5	Squash Salad for Green Lovers	Very Tangy Avocado Cucumber Salad	Steamed Cod Fish With Bizarre Lemon
Day 6	Fancy Broccoli Roasts	Obligatory Yellow Squash Of Magic	Spicy Harissa Infused Magnificent Chicken
Day 7	Squash Salad For Green Lovers	Very Tangy Avocado Cucumber Salad	Steamed Cod Fish With Bizarre Lemon

Reference for Week 3 Shopping List

For Breakfast

Recipe 1: A Bowl of Zucchini Zoodles!

- 2 small sized zucchini
- ½ of an avocado
- ¼ cup of extra virgin olive oil
- 2 tablespoons of water
- 1-2 garlic cloves
- 2 pieces of sweet potatoes
- 2 pieces of whole egg
- 2 tablespoons of green onion
- Salt as needed
- Pepper as needed

Recipe 2: Squash Salad for The Green Lovers!

- 2 tablespoons of extra virgin olive oil
- 1 small sized sliced onion
- 2 medium-sized coarsely chopped tomatoes
- 1 teaspoon of salt
- ¼ teaspoon of pepper
- 2 small zucchini cut up into ½ inch slices
- 2 small sized yellow summer squash cut up into ½ inch slices
- 1 bay leaf
- ½ a teaspoon of dried basil

Recipe 3: Fancy Broccoli Roasts

- 2 heads of broccoli separated into florets
- 2 teaspoons of extra virgin olive oil
- 1 teaspoon of sea salt
- ½ a teaspoon of ground black pepper
- 1 minced garlic clove
- ½ a teaspoon of lemon juice

For Lunch

Recipe 1: Ever so Popular Collard Greens

- 1 tablespoon of extra virgin olive oil

- 3 slices of bacon
- 1 chopped up large onion
- 2 minced garlic cloves
- 1 teaspoon of salt
- 3 cups of chicken broth
- 1 pinch of red pepper flakes
- 1 pound of fresh collard greens cut up into 2 inch pieces

Recipe 2: Very Tangy Avocado and Cucumber Salad

- 2 medium-sized cubed carrots
- 2 cubed avocados
- 4 tablespoons of chopped up fresh cilantro
- 1 minced garlic clove
- 2 tablespoons of minced green onions
- ¼ teaspoon of salt
- Black pepper as needed
- ¼ large sized lemon
- 1 piece of lime

Recipe 3: Obligatory Yellow Squash of Magic

- 4 medium-sized yellow squash
- ½ a cup of extra virgin olive oil
- 2 cloves of crushed garlic
- Salt as needed
- Pepper as needed

For Dinner

Recipe 1: Craziest Tom Ka Gai Ever!

- ¾ pound of skinless, boneless chicken meat
- 3 tablespoons of extra virgin olive oil
- 14 ounce of coconut milk
- 2 cups of water
- 2 tablespoons of minced fresh ginger root
- 4 tablespoons of fish sauce
- ¼ cup of lime juice

- ¼ teaspoon of cayenne pepper
- ½ a teaspoon of turmeric
- 2 tablespoons of thinly sliced green onion
- 1 tablespoon of freshly chopped cilantro

Recipe 2: Steamed Cod Fish With Bizarre Lemon

- 6 ounce of halibut fillets
- 1 tablespoon of dried dill weed
- 1 tablespoon of onion powder
- 2 teaspoons of dried parsley
- ¼ teaspoon of paprika
- 1 pinch of salt
- 1 pinch of lemon pepper
- 1 pinch of garlic powder
- 2 tablespoons of lemon juice

Recipe 3: Spicy Harissa Infused Magnificent Chicken

- 1 large sized egg plant
- 2 tablespoons of extra virgin olive oil
- ¾ pound of organic chicken breast (Cubed up to small sizes)
- 1 chopped up onion
- 2 crushed garlic cloves
- 1 cup of chopped mushrooms
- 2 cups of fresh spinach
- 1 can of diced tomatoes
- 2 tablespoons of Mina Harissa Sauce
- 1 tablespoon of fresh basil
- 1 teaspoon of garlic granules
- Himalayan salt
- Red pepper flakes

Week 4 Meal Plan

Week 4	Breakfast	Lunch	Dinner
Day 1	**Authentic Guacamole!**	**The Constantly Evolving Shrimp Scampi**	**Exotic Kalua Pig!**
Day 2	**The Original Boiled Eggs**	**Herbed up and Cooked Chicken Breast**	**Thinly Braised Balsamic Chicken Ala Gusto!**
Day 3	**Motherly Carrot Soup**	**Rich Guy's Lobster Tails**	**Super Zucchini Soup of Simplicity!**
Day 4	**Authentic Guacamole!**	**The Constantly Evolving Shrimp Scampi**	**Super Zucchini Soup of Simplicity!**
Day 5	**The Original Boiled Eggs**	**Herbed up and Cooked Chicken Breast**	**Exotic Kalua Pig!**
Day 6	**Motherly Carrot Soup**	**Rich Guy's Lobster Tails**	**Thinly Braised Balsamic Chicken Ala Gusto!**
Day 7	**Motherly Carrot Soup**	**Herbed up and Cooked Chicken Breast**	**Super Zucchini Soup of Simplicity!**

Reference for Week 4 Shopping List

For Breakfast

Recipe 1: Authentic Guacamole!

48

- 3 pieces of peeled, mashed and pitted avocado
- 1 juiced lime
- 1 teaspoon of salt
- ½ a cup of diced onion
- 3 tablespoons of chopped fresh cilantro
- 2 diced plum tomatoes
- 1 teaspoon of minced garlic
- 1 pinch of cayenne pepper

Recipe 2: The Original Boiled Eggs

- 1 tablespoon of salt
- ¼ cup of distilled white vinegar
- 6 cups of water
- 8 pieces of eggs

Recipe 3: Motherly Carrot Soup

- 2 tablespoons of extra virgin olive oil
- 1 chopped up onion
- 1 tablespoon of curry powder
- 2 pound of chopped up carrots
- 4 cups of vegetable broth
- 2 cups of water

For Lunch

Recipe 1: The Constantly Evolving Shrimp Scampi

- 4 tablespoons of ghee
- 1 tablespoon of extra virgin olive oil
- 4 minced garlic cloves
- ¼ teaspoon of red pepper flakes
- ¾ pound of shelled and deveined shrimp
- 1 tablespoon of lemon juice
- Zest of ½ a lemon
- 2 tablespoons of freshly minced parsley

Recipe 2: Herbed up Cooked Chicken Breast

- 2 medium sized cubed carrots
- 2 cubed avocados
- 4 tablespoons of chopped up fresh cilantro
- 1 minced garlic clove
- 2 tablespoons of minced green onions
- ¼ teaspoon of salt
- Black pepper as needed
- ¼ large sized lemon
- 1 piece of lime

Recipe 3: Rich Guy's Lobster Tails

- 1 tablespoon of lemon juice
- ½ a cup of extra virgin olive oil
- 1 teaspoon of salt
- 1 teaspoon of paprika
- 1/8 teaspoon of white pepper
- 1/8 teaspoon of garlic powder
- 10 ounce of rock lobster tails

For Dinner

Recipe 1: Exotic Kalua Pig!

- 6 pound of pork butt roast
- 1 and a ½ tablespoon of Hawaiian sea salt
- 1 tablespoon of liquid smoke flavoring

Recipe 2: Thinly Braised Balsamic Chicken Ala Gusto

- 6 boneless, skinless chicken breast halves
- 1 teaspoon of garlic salt
- Ground black pepper as needed
- 2 tablespoons of extra virgin olive oil
- 1 thinly sliced onion
- 1 can of diced tomatoes
- ½ a cup of balsamic vinegar
- 1 teaspoon of dried basil
- 1 teaspoon of dried oregano

- 1 teaspoon of dried rosemary
- ½ a teaspoon of dried thyme

Recipe 3: Super Zucchini Soup of Simplicity

- 2 tablespoons of extra virgin olive oil
- 1 large thinly sliced halved onion
- 1 tablespoon of curry powder
- Salt as needed
- 4 small sized zucchini halved up lengthwise and cut into 1-inch slices
- 1 quart of chicken stock
- 1 cup of chopped mushrooms
- 2 cups of fresh spinach
- 1 can of diced tomatoes
- 2 tablespoons of Mina Harissa Sauce
- 1 tablespoon of fresh basil
- 1 teaspoon of garlic granules
- Himalayan salt
- Red pepper flakes

Week 5 Meal Plan (The Final 2 days)

Week 5	Breakfast	Lunch	Dinner
Day 1	Basic Rattling Acapulco Chicken	Zucchini Pasta for the Millennial	Zinger Soft Calculative Tenderloins
Day 2	Forever Together Courgette Salad	A Darkened Broody Chicken	Amazingly Spicy Pumpkin Chili!

Reference for Week 5 (Final 2 Days) Shopping List

For Breakfast

Recipe 1: Basic Rattling Acapulco Chicken

- 2 skinless and boneless (halved) chicken breasts cut up into bite-sized pieces
- 1 tablespoon of divide chili powder
- Salt as needed
- Pepper as needed
- 1 tablespoon of extra virgin olive oil
- 1 cup of chopped up green bell pepper
- ½ a cup of chopped onion
- 2 jalapeno peppers minced and seeded
- 1 large sized tomato cut up into chunks
- 10 drops of hot pepper sauce

Recipe 2: Forever Together Courgette Salad

- 1 lemon juice
- 2 tablespoons of extra virgin olive oil

- ½ of a small pack of chopped up chives
- ½ of a small chopped up mint
- 300g of courgettes

For Lunch

Recipe 1: A Darkened Broody Chicken

- ½ a teaspoon of paprika
- 1/8 teaspoon of salt
- ¼ teaspoon of cayenne pepper
- ¼ teaspoon of ground cumin
- ¼ teaspoon of dried thyme
- 1/8 teaspoon of ground white pepper
- 1/8 teaspoon of onion powder
- 2 skinless and boneless chicken breast

Recipe 2: Zucchini Pasta for the Millennial

- 2 pieces of peeled Zucchini
- 1 tablespoon of extra virgin olive oil
- ¼ cup of water
- Salt as needed
- Ground black pepper as needed

For Dinner

Recipe 1: Zinger Soft Calculative Tenderloins

- 1 and a ½ cup of fresh lime juice
- ¾ cup of extra virgin olive oil
- 6 sliced garlic cloves
- 2 teaspoons of salt
- 6 tablespoons of dried oregano
- 1 pound of pork tenderloins

Recipe 2: Amazingly Spicy Pumpkin Chili!

- 3 cups of chopped up yellow onion
- 8 cloves of chopped up garlic
- 1 pound of ground turkey
- 2 can of 15-ounce fire roasted tomato
- 2 cups of pumpkin puree
- 1 cup of chicken broth
- 2 tablespoons of honey
- 4 teaspoons of chili spice
- 1 teaspoon of ground cinnamon
- 1 teaspoon of sea salt

Part 3: Finally, the Recipes!

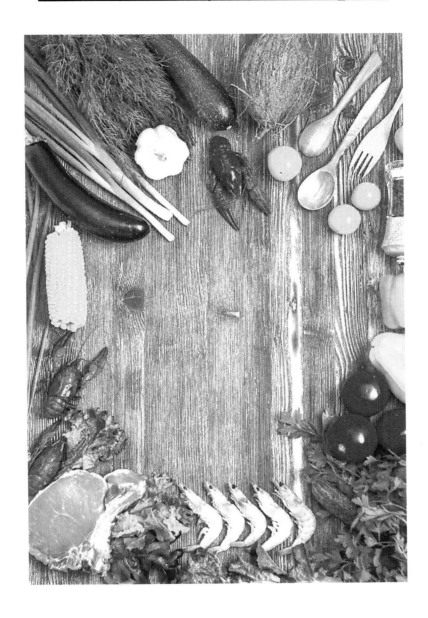

Chapter 9: Breakfast Recipes

BlackBerry and Coconut Chia Pudding

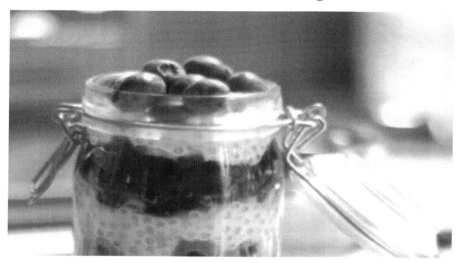

Prep Time: 12 hours

Cooking Time: 0 minute

Serving: 1

Ingredients:

- ½ a cup of blackberries
- 3 tablespoons of chia seeds
- 1 cup of unsweetened almond milk
- ¼ teaspoon of 100% pure vanilla powder
- 1 tablespoon of unsweetened shredded coconut

Directions:

1. Take a small sized mixing bowl and add crushed up blackberries using a fork until a thick jam
2. Add chia seeds, vanilla, shredded coconut and almond milk
3. Stir well and transfer it to a container
4. Once done, allow it to chill overnight

5. Enjoy!

Nutrition:

- Calories: 330
- Fat: 23g
- Carbohydrates: 29g
- Protein: 10g

Sautéed Zucchini for a Refreshing Morning

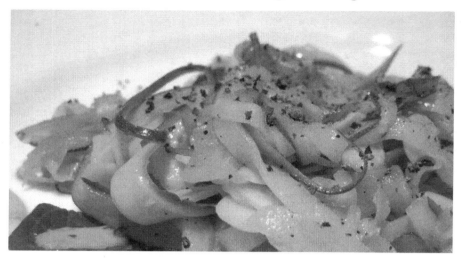

Prep Time: 15 minutes

Cooking Time: 15 minute

Serving: 6

Ingredients:

- 1 tablespoon of extra virgin olive oil
- ½ of a diced red onion
- Salt as needed
- Pepper as needed
- 4 halved and sliced Zucchini
- ½ a pound of fresh sliced mushrooms
- 1 diced tomato
- 1 minced clove of garlic
- 1 teaspoon of Italian seasoning

Directions:

1. Take a large sized skillet and place it over medium heat
2. Add olive oil and allow the oil to heat up
3. Add onions alongside a bit of pepper and Saute the onions for about 2 minutes

4. Stir in mushroom and zucchini
5. Once the Zucchinis are tender, add garlic, Italian seasoning, and tomatoes
6. Cook everything for a few minutes more
7. Enjoy!

Nutrition:

- Calories: 68
- Fat: 4g
- Carbohydrates: 10g
- Protein: 3g

Mesmerizing Poached Eggs

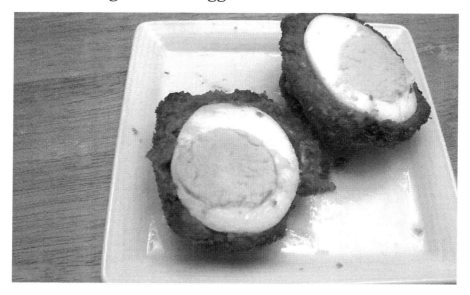

Prep Time: 30 minutes

Cooking Time: 20 minute

Serving: 6

Ingredients:

- 6 medium-sized eggs
- 1 pound of ground pork
- 2 teaspoons of ground cinnamon
- 1-1/2 a teaspoon of salt
- ½ a teaspoon of black pepper
- Ground nutmeg as needed
- Ground clove as needed

Directions:

1. Take a pot and add an inch of water
2. Place the eggs in a steamer basket and allow them to steam for 10 minutes
3. Take a medium bowl and add ice water

4. Once the eggs are done, transfer them to the ice bat hand allow them to cool

5. Peel the eggs

6. Pre-heat your oven to 350 degrees Fahrenheit

7. Take a baking sheet and line it up with parchment paper

8. Take a large sized bowl and add ground pork, salt, pepper

9. Mix well

10. Prepare the scotch egg by taking 1/3 cup of seasoned ground pork and turning it into a lump

11. Flatten the pork into a wide circle like burger patty

12. Put the egg in the center and carefully fold the meat all over

13. Bake for about 15-20 minutes

14. Eat hot!

Nutrition:

- Calories: 330
- Fat: 23g
- Carbohydrates: 29g
- Protein: 10g

Suspenseful and Tangy Potato Sticks

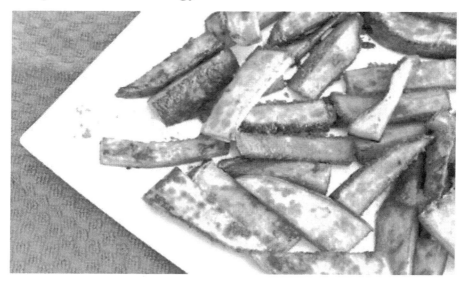

Prep Time: 10 minutes

Cooking Time: 30 minutes

Serving: 2

Ingredients:

- 4 pieces of russet potatoes peeled and cut up into ¼ inch thick fries
- 3 tablespoons of extra virgin olive oil
- 2 tablespoons of lime juice
- 2 garlic cloves minced
- ½ a teaspoon of red pepper flakes
- ¼ teaspoon of cayenne pepper
- 1 teaspoon of chili powder
- 2 tablespoons of spicy brown mustard
- ½ a teaspoon of ground black pepper
- 1 teaspoon of salt

Directions:

1. Pre-heat your oven to a temperature of 400 degrees Fahrenheit
2. Take a large sized bowl and add olive oil, garlic, lime juice, red pepper flakes, cayenne pepper, chili powder, mustard, pepper
3. Mix everything well
4. Add the potatoes slices to the mixture and keep stirring it until the potatoes and nicely coated
5. Arrange the fires in a single layer on your baking sheet
6. Bake for about 20 minutes in your preheated oven
7. Turn the fries over and bake for another 15 minutes until they show a nice crispy texture
8. Season with some salt and pepper
9. Enjoy!

Nutrition:

- Calories: 269
- Fat: 11g
- Carbohydrates: 39g
- Protein: 5g

The Wow-Worthy Extreme Kalamata Olive Tapenade

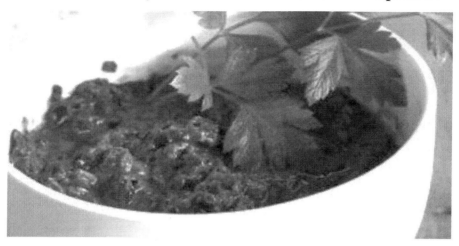

Prep Time: 15 minutes

Cooking Time: 0 minute

Serving: 4

Ingredients:

- 3 peeled garlic cloves
- 1 cup of pitted kalamata olives
- 2 tablespoons of capers
- 3 tablespoons of chopped fresh parsley
- 2 tablespoons of lemon juice
- 2 tablespoons of extra virgin olive oil
- Salt as needed
- Pepper as needed

Directions:

1. Take a food processor and add garlic cloves
2. Pulse them well until they are fully minced
3. Add olives, olive oil, capers, parsley, lemon juice to the food processor and blend them well again until the whole mixture is finely chopped up
4. Season with some pepper and salt to adjust the flavor

5. Serve and enjoy!

Nutrition:

- Calories: 81
- Fat: 8g
- Carbohydrates: 3g
- Protein: 0.5g

Feisty Grilled Artichokes of America

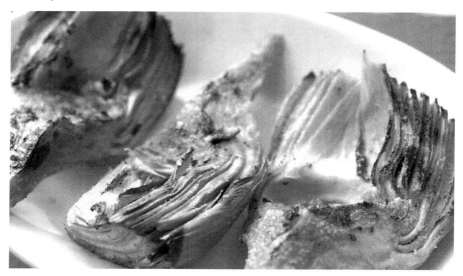

Prep Time: 5 minutes

Cooking Time: 30 minute

Serving: 4

Ingredients:

- 2 large sized artichokes
- 1 quartered lemon
- ¾ cup of extra virgin olive oil
- 4 chopped up garlic cloves
- 1 teaspoon of salt
- ½ a teaspoon of ground black pepper

Directions:

1. Take a large sized bowl and fill it up with cold water

2. Squeeze a bit of lemon juice from the wedges

3. Trim the upper part of your chokes, making sure to trim any damaged leaves as well

4. Cut the chokes up in half lengthwise portions
5. Add the chokes to your bowl of lemon water
6. Bring the whole pot to a boil
7. Pre-heat your outdoor grill to about medium-high heat
8. Allow the chokes to cook in the boiling pot for 15 minutes
9. Drain them the chokes and keep them on the side
10. Take another medium-sized bowl and squeeze the remaining lemon
11. Stir in garlic and olive to the lemon mix
12. Brush up the chokes with the garlic dip and place them on your pre-heated grill
13. Grill for about 10 minutes, making sure to keep basting them until the edges are just slightly charred
14. Serve with the dip and enjoy!

Nutrition:

- Calories: 402
- Fat: 40g
- Carbohydrates: 10g
- Protein: 2.9g

Original Syrian Green Beans Alongside Olive Oil

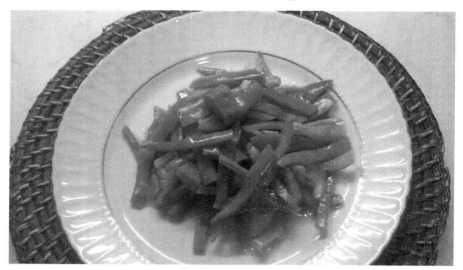

Prep Time: 5 minutes

Cooking Time: 25 minute

Serving: 4

Ingredients:

- 16 ounce of packaged frozen cut green beans
- ¼ cup of extra virgin olive oil
- Salt as needed
- 1 minced garlic clove
- ¼ cup of chopped fresh cilantro leaves

Directions:

1. Take a large sized pot and add the green beans
2. Drizzle olive oil and mix well
3. Season with some salt
4. Cover the pot with a lid and cook the beans over medium-high heat, making sure to keep stirring it from time to time until you have reached your desired consistency

5. Make sure to keep an eye out so that you don't Saute the beans fully but only have a slight brown color
6. Should take about 10-15 minutes
7. Add garlic and cilantro to the beans
8. Cook for another 10 minutes until the cilantro has wilted
9. Serve and enjoy!

Nutrition:

- Calories: 164
- Fat: 14g
- Carbohydrates: 8g
- Protein: 1.6g

The Garlic Kale to Diet for!

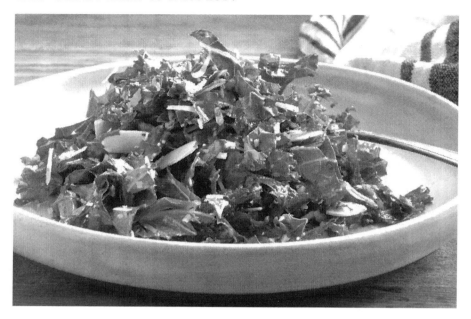

Prep Time: 5 minutes

Cooking Time: 10 minutes

Serving: 4

Ingredients:

- 1 bunch of kale
- 2 tablespoons of extra virgin olive oil
- 4 minced garlic cloves

Directions:

1. Carefully take the kale and tear them into small pieces
2. Toss away the stem as we are not going to need them
3. Take a large sized pot and place it over medium heat
4. Add olive oil and allow it to heat up
5. Add garlic and stir-fry for about 2 minutes until fragrant
6. Add kale and cook for another 5 minutes until the kale shows a bright green color and has wilted

7. Serve hot!

Nutrition:

- Calories: 120
- Fat: 7.5g
- Carbohydrates: 12g
- Protein: 3.9g

Everybody's Favorite Healthy Bok Choy!

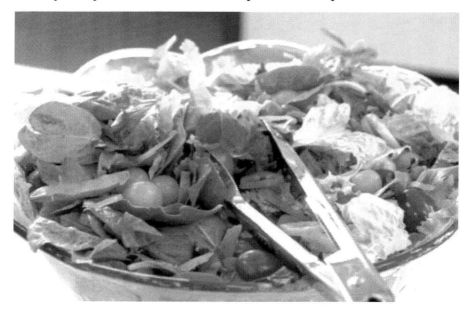

Prep Time: 5 minutes

Cooking Time: 10 minutes

Serving: 4

Ingredients:

- 4 sliced chopped up bacon
- 2 pounds of baby Bok Choy
- 1 teaspoon of extra virgin olive oil
- ½ of a small chopped up red onion
- 1 teaspoon of red pepper flakes
- 1 teaspoon of minced garlic
- Salt as needed

Directions:

1. Take a large sized skillet and place it over medium heat
2. Add the bacon stir fry them until they are browned and crispy

3. Remove the bacon and drain any excess fat (make sure to reserve 1 tablespoon of grease for later use)

4. Add olive oil, garlic, onion and red pepper flakes to the same pan and cook until the onions and soft

5. Add Bok Choy and cover it up with the lid

6. Cook for about 3-5 minutes

7. Remove the lid and cook for another 2 minutes

8. The Bok Choy should now be crispy but tender

9. Stir in bacon

10. Season with some salt

11. Serve immediately!

Nutrition:

- Calories: 97
- Fat: 5.6g
- Carbohydrates: 6g
- Protein: 7g

Surprisingly Cool Omelet Muffins!

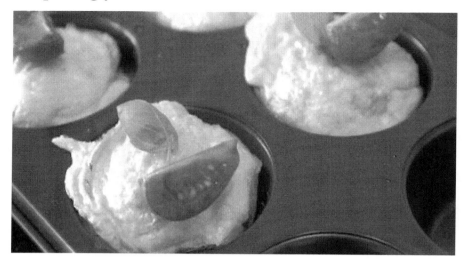

Prep Time: 15 minutes

Cooking Time: 20 minute

Serving: 4

Ingredients:

- 8 pieces of eggs
- 8 ounce of crumbled cooked ham
- 1 cup of diced red bell pepper
- 1 cup of diced onion
- ¼ teaspoon of salt
- 1/8 teaspoon of ground black pepper
- 2 tablespoons of water

Directions:

1. Pre-heat your oven to a temperature of 350 degrees Fahrenheit
2. Take 8 cups of muffin tins and line them up with paper liners
3. Grease them up
4. Take a large sized bowl and beat the eggs

5. Add ham, bell peppers, onion, black pepper, water and salt to the egg mix
6. Pour the egg mix into your muff tins
7. Bake for 20 minutes in your oven
8. Enjoy!

Nutrition:

- Calories: 308
- Fat: 20g
- Carbohydrates: 6.8g
- Protein: 23g

Suspenseful BLT Egg Salad

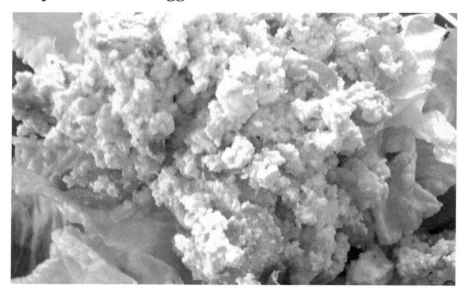

Prep Time: 10 minutes

Cooking Time: 10 minute

Serving: 4

Ingredients:

- 1 piece of avocado
- 6 pieces of hardboiled egg
- ¾ cup of grape tomatoes cut up into halves
- 4 strips of bacon cooked crispy
- ½ a cup of chopped green onion
- 2 teaspoons of garlic powder
- ½ a teaspoon of sea salt

Directions:

1. Prepare the hard-boiled eggs (following the provided recipe in the book)
2. Take skillet and place it over medium heat
3. Add the bacon and cook them until crispy

4. Take a medium bowl and add the cooked (peeled up) eggs, avocado, salt and garlic

5. Smash everything well using a fork

6. Add cooked bacon pieces, scallions, and tomatoes

7. Mix well

8. Taste and season it with ground garlic and salt

9. Serve with spinach or inside beautiful lettuce wraps

10. Enjoy!

Nutrition:

- Calories: 250
- Fat: 16g
- Carbohydrates: 4g
- Protein: 12g

Authentic Whole Foods Compliant Baked Egg

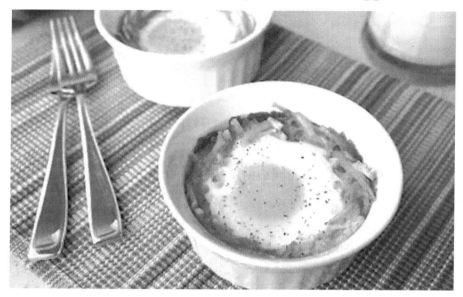

Prep Time: 10 minutes

Cooking Time: 30 minutes

Serving: 4

Ingredients:

- 1 cup of water
- 1 cup of marinara sauce
- 4 pieces of eggs

Directions:

1. Pre-heat your oven to a temperature of 350 degrees Fahrenheit
2. Take a kettle and pour water into it
3. Heat up the kettle until steaming
4. Remove the heat and pour about 1 cup of the steaming water into the bottom of a casserole dish
5. Take 2-3 ramekins
6. Pour ¼ cup of marinara sauce into each of your ramekins
7. Crack 1 egg into the ramekins

8. Arrange the ramekins in your casserole dish

9. Fill up the dish with enough water to reach about the midpoint of the ramekin

10. Bake for about 25 minutes until the yolks are firm

11. Serve and enjoy!

Nutrition:

- Calories: 126
- Fat: 6.7g
- Carbohydrates: 9g
- Protein: 7.4g

Feisty Banana Chia Pudding!

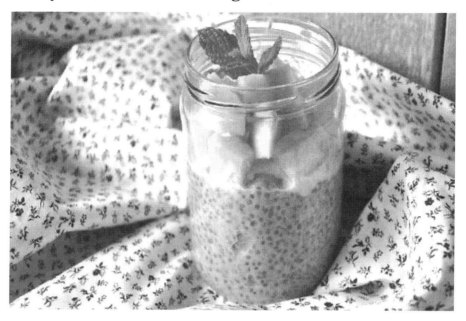

Prep Time: 40 minutes

Cooking Time: 0 minute

Serving: 4

Ingredients:

- 1 cup of water
- 2 and a ½ tablespoon of Chia Seeds
- 2 Ripe pieces of Bananas
- 1 cup of Full Fat Coconut Milk
- ½ a teaspoon of Ground Cinnamon
- Just a pinch of salt

Directions:

1. Take a pint jar and add water and chia seeds
2. Lock it tight and give it a shake
3. Keep it on the side for 30 minutes

4. Take a food processor and add bananas, coconut milk and pulse well
5. Pour the banana mix into your quart-sized bowl
6. Add in the previously prepared chia mix alongside chia gel and salt
7. Store in your fridge and allow it to chill
8. Enjoy!

Nutrition:

- Calories: 134
- Fat: 9g
- Carbohydrates: 12g
- Protein: 2g

The Irish Bacon and Cabbage Soup

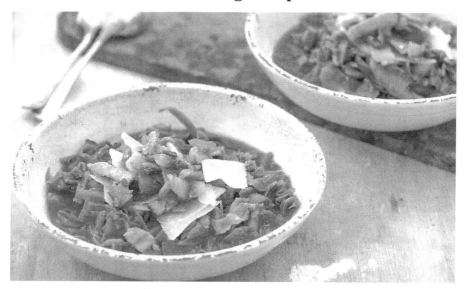

Prep Time: 15 minutes

Cooking Time: 30 minutes

Serving: 4

Ingredients:

- ½ a pound of Irish bacon (diced up)
- 2 large sized peeled and cubed potatoes
- 15 ounce of diced tomatoes with juice
- 1 cup of chicken stock
- Salt as needed
- Pepper as needed
- 2 cups of thinly sliced dark green Savoy cabbage leaves

Directions:

1. Take a large sized saucepan/pot and place it over medium-high heat

2. Cook the bacon until it is nicely browned on all sides

3. Drain any excess fat

4. Stir in potatoes, chicken stock and tomatoes to the pot and cover up the bacon
5. Season with some salt and pepper
6. Bring the whole mixture to a boil
7. Lower down the heat immediately once boiling point has been reached
8. Allow it to simmer for 20 minutes
9. Stir in cabbage and allow it to simmer for a few minutes more
10. Serve hot!

Nutrition:

- Calories: 276
- Fat: 8g
- Carbohydrates: 38g
- Protein: 12g

Whole Foods appreciated Cinnamon Coffee

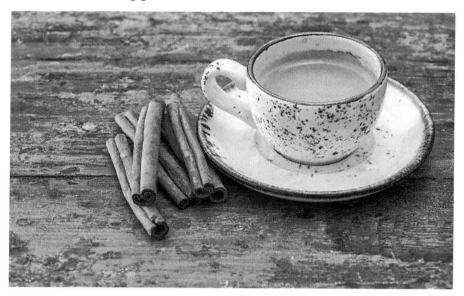

Prep Time: 5 minutes

Cooking Time: 10 minutes

Serving: 2

Ingredients:

- 2 tablespoons of ground coffee
- 1 teaspoon of ground cinnamon
- 10 ounce of hot water

Directions:

1. Take a small sized bowl and add cinnamon and coffee
2. Pour hot water into the bowl
3. Allow it to brew for about 5 minutes
4. Strain the coffee into your favorite coffee mug
5. Enjoy!

Nutrition:

- Calories: 12
- Fat: 0g
- Carbohydrates: 3g
- Protein: 0.4g

Melodious Artichoke Salsa

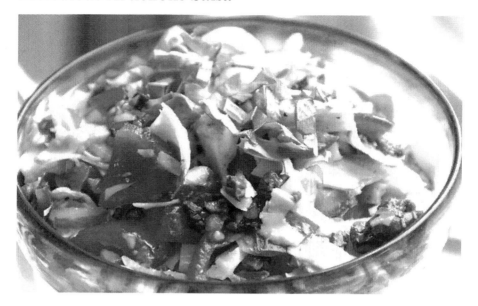

Prep Time: 10 minutes

Cooking Time: 0 minute

Serving: 32

Ingredients:

- 6.5 ounce of drained artichoke hearts (chopped)
- 3 chopped up plum tomatoes
- 2 tablespoons of chopped up red onion
- ¼ cup of chopped up black olives
- 1 tablespoon of chopped up garlic
- 2 tablespoons of chopped up fresh basil
- Salt as needed
- Pepper as needed

Directions:

1. Take a medium-sized bowl and add artichoke hearts, onion, and tomatoes
2. Mix well and add garlic, olives, tomatoes and mix again

3. Season with some salt and pepper according to your preference
4. Serve chilled with your favorite tortilla chips!

Nutrition:

- Calories: 52
- Fat: 3g
- Carbohydrates: 7g
- Protein: 2g

Unapologetic Tomatillo Salsa Verde

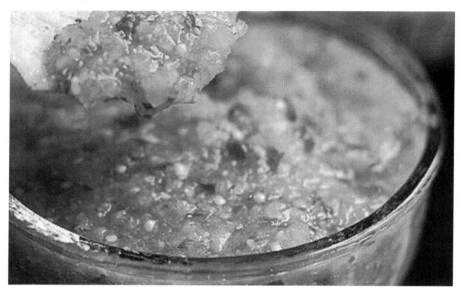

Prep Time: 10 minutes

Cooking Time: 15 minutes

Serving: 24

Ingredients:

- 1 and a ½ pound of tomatillos
- ½ - 1 piece of jalapeno
- 1 poblano pepper
- ½ of a white onion cut up into ¼ portions
- 1 halved Roma tomato
- 2 cloves of peeled garlic
- ¼-1/2 a cup of cilantro
- 1 and a ½ teaspoon of white vinegar
- ½ a teaspoon of salt

Directions:

1. Pre-heat your broiler

2. Take a baking sheet and add jalapeno, tomatillos, poblano pepper and onion

3. Broil until nicely blackened

4. Turn them with tong if needed

5. Remove them from the broiler and allow them to cool

6. Pull off the stem from the poblano and deseed it

7. Discard

8. Transfer the tomatillo, jalapeno, poblano, Roma tomato, cilantro, garlic and white vinegar to a food processor

9. Season with some salt

10. Process well until a nice texture appears

11. Season with some more salt if needed

12. Enjoy!

Nutrition:

- Calories: 24
- Fat: 0.6g
- Carbohydrates: 4.6g
- Protein: 0.8g

Very Refreshing Tomato Salsa

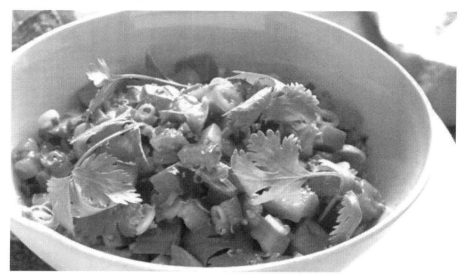

Prep Time: 10 minutes

Cooking Time: 10 minutes

Serving: 24

Ingredients:

- 12 Roma tomatoes
- 2 unpeeled garlic cloves
- 1 quartered small onion
- 1 jalapeno Chile pepper
- 1 and a ½ tablespoon of extra virgin olive oil
- 1 teaspoon of ground cumin
- ¼ teaspoon of salt
- 3 tablespoons of fresh lime juice
- ¼ cup of chopped fresh cilantro

Directions:

1. Prepare your broiler by pre-heating it up
2. Take a medium-sized baking dish and add onion, jalapeno, Roma tomatoes, garlic and Chile pepper

3. Drizzle the veggies with olive oil

4. Boil for about 5-10 minutes until the vegetables are charred

5. Remove the heat

6. Discard the tomato cores, garlic skins and jalapeno stems

7. Add vegetables to your food processor and blend it until you get a coarse texture

8. Transfer the mix to a medium-sized bowl and add salt, cumin, cilantro and lime juice

9. Serve the salsa with alone or with your favorite dipper!

Nutrition:

- Calories: 16
- Fat:0.9g
- Carbohydrates: 1.8g
- Protein: 0.4g

Motherly Carrot Soup

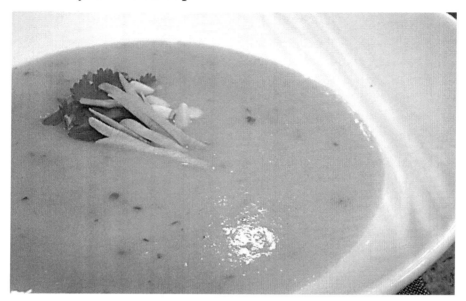

Prep Time: 15 minutes

Cooking Time: 25 minutes

Serving: 24

Ingredients:

- 2 tablespoons of extra virgin olive oil
- 1 chopped up onion
- 1 tablespoon of curry powder
- 2 pound of chopped up carrots
- 4 cups of vegetable broth
- 2 cups of water

Directions:

1. Take a large sized pot and place it over medium heat
2. Add oil and allow it to heat up
3. Add onions and Saute until translucent
4. Stir in curry powder and chopped up carrots

5. Keep stirring well until the carrots are finely coated

6. Pour vegetable broth into the pot and allow it to simmer for 20 minutes until the carrots are tender

7. Transfer the whole mixture to a blender and blend until a smooth puree forms

8. Pour the puree back into the pot

9. Add a bit of water to adjust the consistency

10. Warm it and enjoy!

Nutrition:

- Calories: 133
- Fat: 5.4g
- Carbohydrates: 20g
- Protein: 2.4g

The Original Boiled Egg

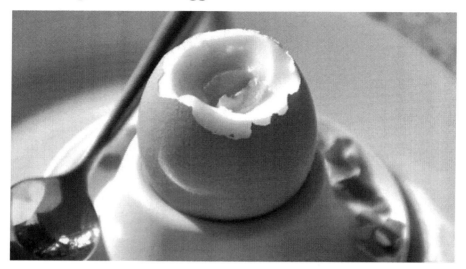

Prep Time: 5 minutes

Cooking Time: 20 minutes

Serving: 8

Ingredients:

- 1 tablespoon of salt
- ¼ cup of distilled white vinegar
- 6 cups of water
- 8 pieces of eggs

Directions:

1. Take a large sized pot and add salt, vinegar and water
2. Bring the pot to a boil and place it over high heat
3. Add one egg to the pot at a time
4. Bring it to a boil and lower down the heat to a gentle boil
5. Cook for about 14 minutes
6. Once den remove the eggs from the water and place them in a container with cold water
7. Allow it to cool for 15 minutes

8. Peel the eggs and enjoy!

Nutrition:

- Calories: 72
- Fat: 5g
- Carbohydrates: 0.4g
- Protein: 6.3g

Corned Beef Hash for the Coming Age

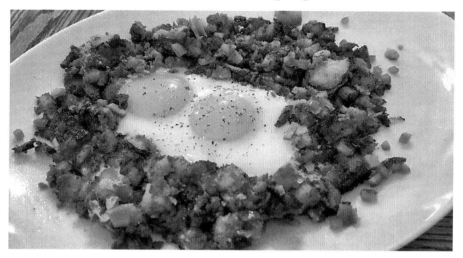

Prep Time: 10 minutes

Cooking Time: 30 minute

Serving: 6

Ingredients:

- 6 pieces of peeled and diced potatoes
- 12 ounce of corned beef chunks
- 1 chopped up medium onion
- 1 cup of beef broth

Directions:

1. Take a large sized deep skillet and place it over medium heat
2. Add potatoes, beef broth, corned beef and onion
3. Cover it up and allow it to simmer for 30 minutes until the potatoes are tender and the liquid has evaporated
4. Give the whole meal a nice mixture
5. Serve and enjoy!

Nutrition:

- Calories: 434
- Fat: 9g
- Carbohydrates: 66g
- Protein: 23g

Very Slowly Baked "Volcanic" Potatoes

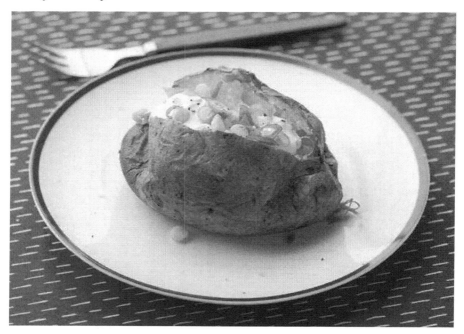

Prep Time: 10 minutes

Cooking Time: 4 hours and 30 minutes

Serving: 4

Ingredients:

- 4 pieces of baking potatoes
- 1 tablespoon of extra virgin olive oil
- Kosher salt as needed
- 4 sheets of aluminum foil

Directions:

11. Take a fork and gently prick your potatoes multiple times
12. Rub the potato all over with olive oil
13. Season the potato with salt
14. Carefully wrap the potato tightly using aluminum foil

15. Place the wrapped up potato in your slow cooker and cook for about 4 and a ½ hour on HIGH settings
16. Once done, gently carve the center and split
17. Garnish with some additional seasoning or mix-ins if you need
18. Enjoy!

Nutrition:

- Calories: 254
- Fat: 4g
- Carbohydrates: 51g
- Protein: 6g

Chicken and Mango Mixture of Creativity

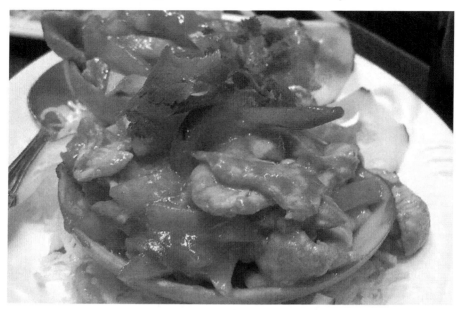

Prep Time: 25 minutes

Cooking Time: 10 minutes

Serving: 4

Ingredients:

- 2 medium-sized peeled and sliced mangoes
- 10 ounce of coconut milk
- 4 teaspoons of extra virgin olive oil
- 4 teaspoons of spicy curry paste
- 14 ounce of skinless and boneless chicken breast halves cut up into cubes
- 4 medium-sized shallots
- 1 large sized English cucumber (seeded and sliced)

Directions:

1. Slice up half of your mangoes and add the halves to a bowl
2. Add the mangoes to a blender alongside coconut milk and blend until a smooth consistency appears
3. Keep the mixture on the side
4. Take a large sized pot and place it over medium-high heat
5. Add oil and allow the oil to heat up
6. Add curry paste and cook for about 1 minute until a calming fragrance appears
7. Add shallots and chicken pieces to the pot and cook for about 5 minutes until the chicken is soft and shallots are tender
8. Pour the mango puree into the mixture and allow it to heat up
9. Serve the mixture with mango slices and cucumbers
10. Stir it and enjoy!

Nutrition:

- Calories: 398
- Fat: 20g
- Carbohydrates: 31g
- Protein: 26g

A Very Mean and Red Chili Beef

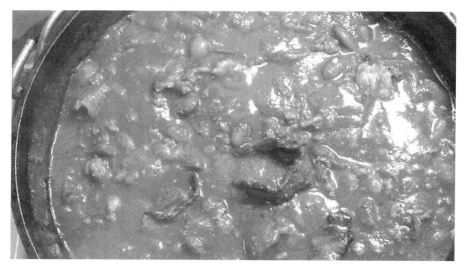

Prep Time: 15 minutes

Cooking Time: 60 minute

Serving: 6

Ingredients:

- 1 pound of ground beef
- 2 minced garlic cloves
- 1 chopped large onion
- 2 tablespoons of chili powder
- 1 teaspoon of dried oregano
- 1 teaspoon of ground cumin
- 1 teaspoon of hot pepper sauce
- 28 ounce of crushed tomatoes
- ¼ cup of red wine vinegar

Directions:

1. Take a large sized stock pot and add your crumbled ground beef

2. Place it over medium-high heat

3. Add garlic and onion to the pot and cook until the beef is properly cooked

4. Season with some chili powder, hot sauce, cumin and oregano

5. Stir in tomatoes and vinegar and bring the whole mixture to a boil

6. Lower down the heat and simmer for 1 hour

7. Stir from time to time to ensure that it does not burn

8. Serve and enjoy!

Nutrition:

- Calories: 226
- Fat: 12g
- Carbohydrates: 14g
- Protein: 15g

Slightly Spicy Medley of Mango and Salsa

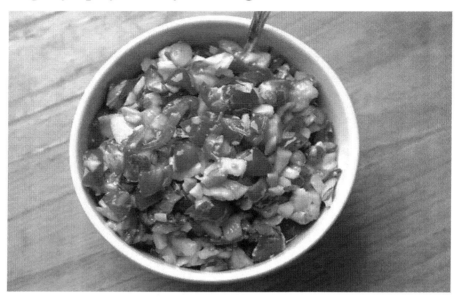

Prep Time: 10 minutes

Cooking Time: 30 minutes

Serving: 6

Ingredients:

- 1 peeled and deseeded mango (sliced)
- 1 peeled, pitted and diced avocado
- 4 medium sized diced tomatoes
- 1 deseeded and minced jalapeno pepper
- ½ a cup of chopped up fresh cilantro
- 3 minced garlic cloves
- 1 teaspoon of salt
- 2 tablespoons of fresh lime juice
- ¼ cup of chopped red onion
- 3 tablespoons of extra virgin olive oil

Directions:

1. Take a medium-sized bowl and add avocado, tomatoes, mango, garlic, jalapeno, cilantro and mix everything well
2. Stir in salt, red onion, olive oil and lime juice
3. Mix well
4. Chill it in your fridge for about 30 minutes to allow the flavors to blend in
5. Enjoy solo or as s dipping!

Nutrition:

- Calories: 158
- Fat: 12g
- Carbohydrates: 13g
- Protein: 1.9g

Astonishing Baked Avocado Eggs

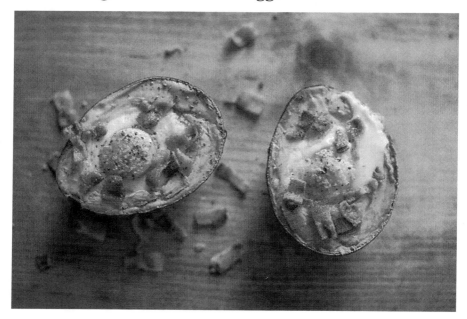

Prep Time: 5 minutes

Cooking Time: 15 minute

Serving: 4

Ingredients:

- 2 pieces of eggs
- 1 piece of avocado
- ½ of a squeeze lemon
- Salt as needed
- Pepper as needed

Directions:

1. Pre-heat your oven to a temperature of 425 degrees Fahrenheit
2. Scoop out the flesh off your avocado leaving about ½ an inch of avocado rim
3. Break an egg into the avocado

106

4. Place it on your baking sheet
5. Sprinkle lemon juice, pepper, salt over your avocado halves
6. Bake for about 15 minutes until the yolks are set
7. Enjoy once done!

Nutrition:

- Calories: 134
- Fat: 9g
- Carbohydrates: 12g
- Protein: 2g

A Bowl of Zucchini Zoodles!

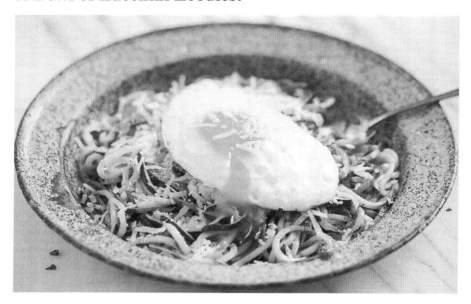

Prep Time: 15 minutes

Cooking Time: 15 minute

Serving: 2

Ingredients:

- 2 small sized zucchini
- ½ of an avocado
- ¼ cup of extra virgin olive oil
- 2 tablespoons of water
- 1-2 garlic cloves
- 2 pieces of sweet potatoes
- 2 pieces of whole egg
- 2 tablespoons of green onion
- Salt as needed
- Pepper as needed

Directions:

1. Remove the skin off your sweet potatoes and chop them up into bite-sized portions
2. Take a skillet and place it over medium-high heat
3. Add 2 tablespoons of olive oil and allow it to heat up
4. Add potatoes and cook them
5. Chop up the end of your zucchini and pass them through a Spiralizer to turn them into zoodles
6. Keep the zoodles on the side
7. Prepare your avocado cream by taking a bowl and adding 2 tablespoons of olive oil, garlic, avocado and water
8. Mix well
9. Transfer the mixture to your food processor and pulse well
10. Give it a nice stir and pour the mixture over your zoodles
11. Add cooked potatoes on top of the zoodles as well
12. Mix well
13. Cook 2 eggs and transfer them on top of your zoodles
14. Garnish with some pepper ,salt and onion
15. Mix well and serve!

Nutrition:

- Calories: 228
- Fat: 12g
- Carbohydrates: 16g
- Protein: 17g

Squash Salad for the Green Lovers!

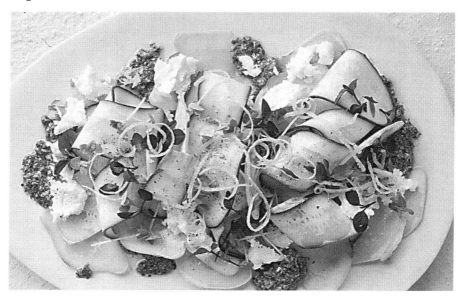

Prep Time: 15 minutes

Cooking Time: 30 minutes

Serving: 4

Ingredients:

- 2 tablespoons of extra virgin olive oil
- 1 small sized sliced onion
- 2 medium-sized coarsely chopped tomatoes
- 1 teaspoon of salt
- ¼ teaspoon of pepper
- 2 small zucchini cut up into ½ inch slices
- 2 small sized yellow summer squash cut up into ½ inch slices
- 1 bay leaf
- ½ a teaspoon of dried basil

Directions:

1. Take a skillet and place it over medium heat
2. Add oil and allow it to heat up

3. Add onions and stir-fry them for about 5 minutes

4. Add tomatoes to the pan and mix well

5. Season the mixture with salt and pepper

6. Keep stirring for about 5 minutes until nicely cooked

7. Add bay leaf, zucchini, yellow squash, basil and allow it to cover it up

8. Lower down the heat and allow it to simmer for about 20 minutes, making sure to keep stirring it occasionally

9. Discard the bay leaf and enjoy!

Nutrition:

- Calories: 65
- Fat:5g
- Carbohydrates: 5g
- Protein: 1.5g

Fancy Broccoli Roasts

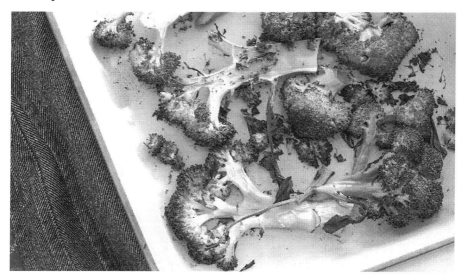

Prep Time: 10 minutes

Cooking Time: 15 minutes

Serving: 6

Ingredients:

- 2 heads of broccoli separated into florets
- 2 teaspoons of extra virgin olive oil
- 1 teaspoon of sea salt
- ½ a teaspoon of ground black pepper
- 1 minced garlic clove
- ½ a teaspoon of lemon juice

Directions:

1. Preheat your oven to a temperature of 400 degrees Fahrenheit
2. Take a large sized bowl and add broccoli florets
3. Add extra virgin olive oil, sea salt, garlic, and pepper
4. Toss well and mix
5. Spread the broccoli out in a single layer on your baking sheet

6. Bake in your oven for about 20 minutes until the florets are tender and soft enough to be pierced using a fork
7. Squeeze lemon juice on top generously
8. Serve and enjoy!

Nutrition:

- Calories: 49
- Fat: 1.9g
- Carbohydrates: 7g
- Protein: 2.9g

Fresh Avocado and Cilantro Bowl

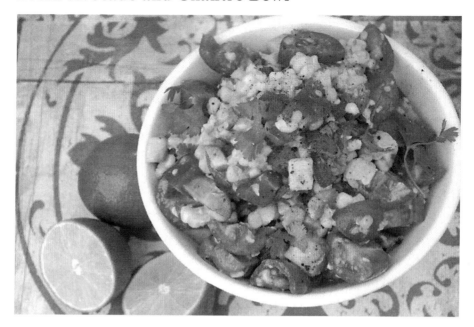

Prep Time: 10 minutes

Cooking Time: 0 minute

Serving: 6

Ingredients:

- 2 avocados – peeled, pitted and diced
- 1 chopped up sweet onion
- 1 green bell pepper (chopped up)
- 1 large sized chopped up ripe tomato
- ¼ cup of chopped up fresh cilantro
- ½ of a juiced lime
- Salt as needed
- Pepper as needed

Directions:

1. Take a medium-sized bowl and add the avocados onion, tomato, bell pepper, cilantro and lime juice
2. Give the whole mixture a nice toss to ensure that everything is coated well with the juice
3. Season with some additional salt and pepper if needed
4. Enjoy!

Nutrition:

- Calories: 126
- Fat: 10g
- Carbohydrates: 10g
- Protein: 2.1g

Ever so Popular Collard Greens

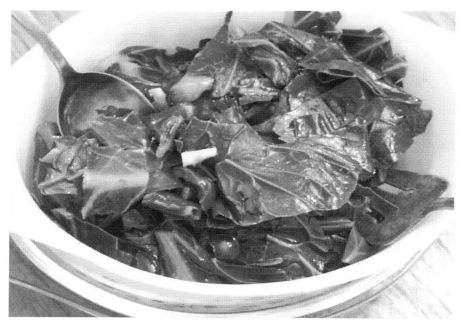

Prep Time: 10 minutes

Cooking Time: 1 hour

Serving: 6

Ingredients:

- 1 tablespoon of extra virgin olive oil
- 3 slices of bacon
- 1 chopped up large onion
- 2 minced garlic cloves
- 1 teaspoon of salt
- 3 cups of chicken broth
- 1 pinch of red pepper flakes
- 1 pound of fresh collard greens cut up into 2 inch pieces

Directions:

1. Take a large sized pan and place it over medium-high heat
2. Pour oil and allow it to heat up
3. Add bacon and cook until crispy and browned
4. Remove the bacon from the pan and crumble it
5. Return the crumbled bacon to the pan again
6. Add onions and cook for 5 minutes
7. Add garlic and cook until fragrant
8. Add collard greens and keep frying until they wilt
9. Pour chicken broth
10. Season with some pepper, red pepper flakes and salt
11. Lower down the heat to low and simmer for 45 minutes
12. Serve hot once done!

Nutrition:

- Calories: 127
- Fat: 9.2g
- Carbohydrates: 7.9g
- Protein: 4.4g

Authentic Guacamole!

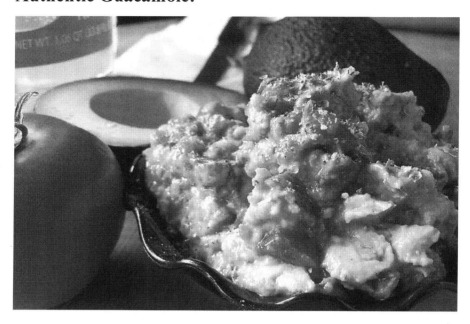

Prep Time: 10 minutes

Cooking Time: 0 minute

Serving: 4

Ingredients:

- 3 pieces of peeled, mashed and pitted avocado
- 1 juiced lime
- 1 teaspoon of salt
- ½ a cup of diced onion
- 3 tablespoons of chopped fresh cilantro
- 2 diced plum tomatoes
- 1 teaspoon of minced garlic
- 1 pinch of cayenne pepper

Directions:

1. Taker a medium-sized bowl and add avocados, salt, and lime juice
2. Mash everything well
3. Stir in onion, cilantro and tomatoes
4. Mix well
5. Add cayenne pepper for a bit of spice
6. Allow it to chill for about an hour
7. Enjoy!

Nutrition:

- Calories: 262
- Fat: 22.2g
- Carbohydrates: 18g
- Protein: 3.7g

Mouthwatering Eastern Chakchouka

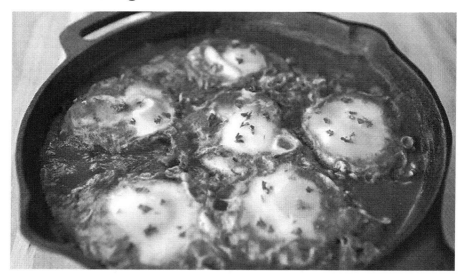

Prep Time: 20 minutes

Cooking Time: 20 minute

Serving: 4

Ingredients:

- 3 tablespoons of extra virgin olive oil
- 1 and a 1/3 cup of chopped up onions
- 1 cup of thinly sliced bell peppers
- 2 minced garlic cloves
- 2 and a ½ cups of chopped tomatoes
- 1 teaspoon of ground cumin
- 1 teaspoon of paprika
- 1 teaspoon of salt
- 1 hot chili pepper finely chopped and deseeded
- 4 pieces of eggs

Directions:

1. Take a skillet and place it over medium heat
2. Pour olive oil and allow it to heat up

3. Stir in garlic, onions, bell pepper to the pan and Saute for about 5 minutes until the onions and tender and translucent

4. Take a bowl and add cumin, salt, tomatoes, chile pepper

5. Mix well

6. Pour tomato mix into your skillet and keep stirring well

7. Simmer for about 10 minutes (uncovered) until the mixture is cooked

8. Make four indents using your finger and crack an egg into each of the indents

9. Cover the skillet and cook for another 5 minutes

10. Serve hot!

Nutrition:

- Calories: 209
- Fat: 15g
- Carbohydrates: 12g
- Protein: 7.8g

Chapter 10: Lunch Recipes

A Very Healthy Cabbage Soup

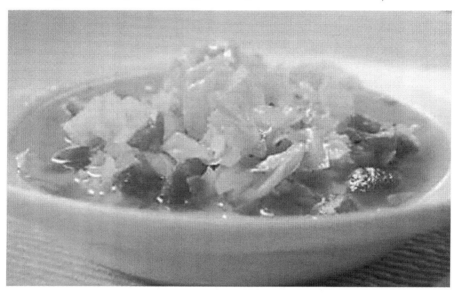

Prep Time: 30 minutes

Cooking Time: 45 minutes

Serving: 8

Ingredients:

- 3 tablespoons of extra virgin olive oil
- ½ of a chopped onion
- 2 chopped garlic cloves
- 2 quarts of water
- 4 cups of chicken broth
- 1 teaspoon of salt
- ½ a teaspoon of black pepper
- ½ of a cabbage head (chopped and cored)
- 14 ounce of drained and diced tomatoes

Directions:

1. Take a large pot and place it over medium heat
2. Add olive oil and allow it to heat up
3. Stir in garlic, onion and cook for about 5 minutes
4. Stir in water, bouillon, salt, and pepper
5. Bring the whole mixture to a boil and stir in cabbage
6. Lower down the heat and simmer for about 10 minutes
7. Stir in tomatoes and return the mix to boil again
8. Lower down the heat and simmer for another 15-30 minutes
9. Stir and serve well!

Nutrition:

- Calories: 92
- Fat: 5.2g
- Carbohydrates: 8.6g
- Protein: 1.5g

Law Breaking Simple Asparagus

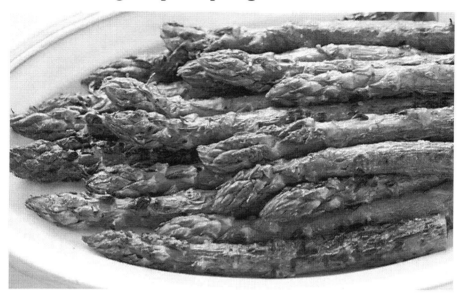

Prep Time: 15 minutes

Cooking Time: 3 minutes

Serving: 2

Ingredients:

- 1 pound of trimmed asparagus
- 1 tablespoon of extra virgin olive oil
- Salt as needed
- Pepper as needed

Directions:

1. Prepare your grill by preheating it to High-Heat
2. Coat the asparagus carefully with olive oil and season them well with pepper and salt
3. Grill for about 3 minutes over high heat
4. Serve and enjoy!

Nutrition:

- Calories: 53
- Fat: 3.5g
- Carbohydrates: 4.4g
- Protein: 2.5g

Surprisingly Healthy Broccoli Soup

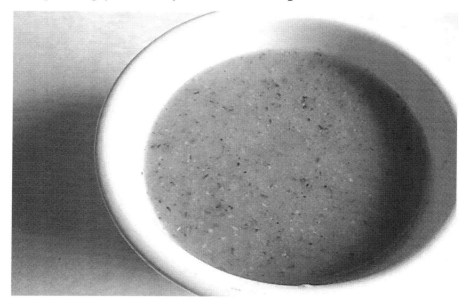

Prep Time: 15 minutes

Cooking Time: 25 minutes

Serving: 6

Ingredients:

- 1 tablespoon of extra virgin olive oil
- 1 chopped-up large onion
- 3 peeled and chopped garlic
- 10 ounce of frozen broccoli
- 1 peeled and chopped potato
- 4 cups of chicken broth
- ¼ teaspoon of ground nutmeg
- Salt as needed
- Pepper as needed

Directions:

1. Take a large sized saucepan and carefully place it over medium heat
2. Add olive oil and allow it to heat up
3. Add garlic and onion and Saute them well until a soft texture appears
4. Add potato, broccoli, and chicken broth
5. Bring the mix to a boil and immediately lower down the heat once boiling point reaches
6. Allow it to simmer for 15 minutes until the veggies are tender
7. Take a blender and puree the whole mixture
8. Return the mix to your saucepan and re-heat for a while
9. Season with some salt, pepper, and nutmeg. Serve and enjoy!

Nutrition:

- Calories: 206
- Fat:12g
- Carbohydrates: 18g
- Protein: 8g

Sun-Dancing Mysterious Aloo Gobi

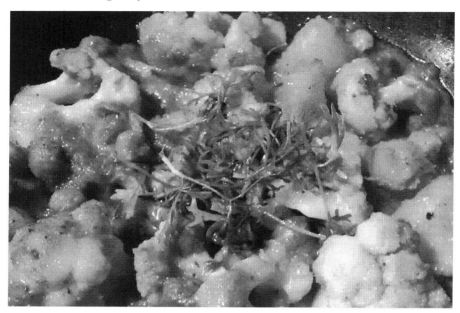

Prep Time: 15 minutes

Cooking Time: 20 minutes

Serving: 2

Ingredients:

- 1 tablespoon of extra virgin olive oil
- 1 teaspoon of cumin seeds
- 1 teaspoon of minced garlic
- 1 teaspoon of ginger paste
- 2 medium-sized peeled and cubed potatoes
- ½ a teaspoon of ground turmeric
- ½ a teaspoon of paprika
- 1 teaspoon of ground cumin
- ½ a teaspoon of Garam masala
- Salt as needed
- 1 pound of cauliflower
- 1 teaspoon of chopped fresh cilantro

Directions:

1. Take a medium-sized skillet and place it over medium heat
2. Add oil and heat it up
3. Add cumin seeds, garlic and ginger paste
4. Cook for about 1 minute until the garlic has been lightly browned up and releases fragrant
5. Add potatoes and season with turmeric, paprika, Garam Masala, salt and cumin
6. Cover the skillet and cook for 5-7 minutes
7. Add cauliflower, cilantro
8. Lower down the heat and stir for 10 minutes (making sure to keep stirring it)
9. Once done, enjoy!

Nutrition:

- Calories: 135
- Fat:4g
- Carbohydrates: 23g
- Protein: 4g

Uncle Adam's Turkey Vegetables!

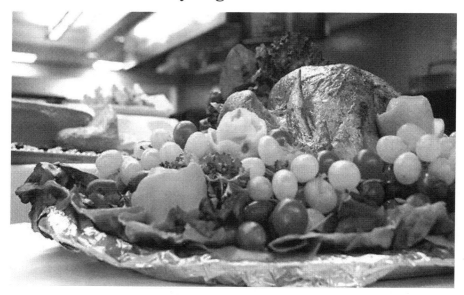

Prep Time: 20 minutes

Cooking Time: 30 minutes

Serving: 4

Ingredients:

- 4 green bell pepper with tops removed and deseeded
- 1 pound of ground turkey
- 2 tablespoons of extra virgin olive oil
- 1/2 of a chopped onion
- 1 cup of sliced mushroom
- 1 chopped up zucchini
- ½ of a red chopped bell pepper
- ½ of a yellow chopped bell pepper
- 1 cup of fresh spinach
- 14 ounce of drained tomatoes
- 1 tablespoon of tomato paste
- Italian seasoning
- Garlic as needed

- Salt as needed
- Pepper as needed

Directions:

1. Pre-heat your oven to a temperature of 350 degrees Fahrenheit
2. Wrap up the green bell peppers in aluminum foil and place them in your baking dish
3. Bake for about 15 minutes
4. Remove the heat
5. Take a skillet and carefully place it over medium heat
6. Add the turkey and cook them until all side has been evenly browned
7. Keep it on the side
8. Pour oil into the skillet and allow it to heat up
9. Add zucchini, onion, mushrooms, spinach, red bell pepper, yellow bell pepper and cook until everything is tender
10. Return the cooked turkey to the skillet
11. Add tomatoes and tomato paste
12. Season with garlic powder, pepper, salt and Italian seasoning
13. Cook well and stuff the green peppers with the mixture
14. Return the peppers to your oven and bake for another 15 minutes
15. Serve and enjoy!

Nutrition:

- Calories: 280
- Fat: 15g
- Carbohydrates: 10.2g
- Protein: 25g

Pretentious Kielbasa and Peppered Potatoes

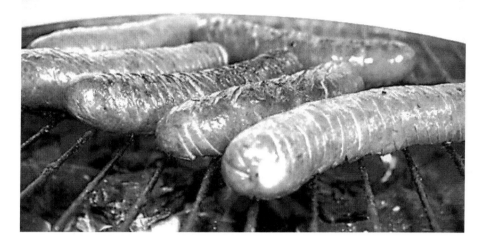

Prep Time: 10 minutes

Cooking Time: 30 minutes

Serving: 6

Ingredients:

- 1 tablespoon of extra virgin olive oil
- 15 ounce of package smoked kielbasa sausage all diced up
- 6 medium sized diced red potatoes
- 1 sliced red bell pepper
- 1 sliced yellow bell pepper

Directions:

1. Take skillet or saucepan and place it over medium heat
2. Add oil and allow it to heat up
3. Add sausages and potatoes and cook for about 25 minutes (covered)
4. Keep stirring it

5. Add yellow and red peppers to the pan
6. Keep cooking for about 5 minutes until the peppers are soft
7. Serve and enjoy!

Nutrition:

- Calories: 404
- Fat: 23g
- Carbohydrates: 36g
- Protein: 13g

Gently Smothered Green Beans Of Delight!

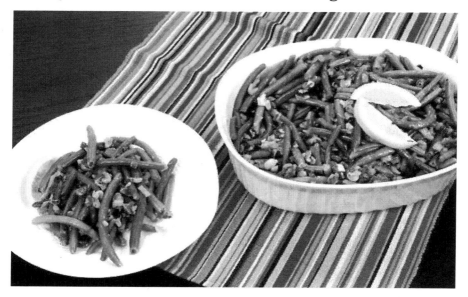

Prep Time: 15 minutes

Cooking Time: 25 minutes

Serving: 6

Ingredients:

- 6 thick slices of chopped bacon
- ½ a cup of minced onion
- 1 teaspoon of minced garlic
- 1 pound of trimmed fresh green beans
- 1 cup of water
- 1/8 teaspoon of salt
- 1 pinch of ground black pepper

Directions:

1. Take a large sized skillet and place it over medium-high heat
2. Add bacon and cook them well
3. Keep the grease on the side and drain them
4. Stir in garlic, onion and cook for 1 minute more

5. Add water and beans and allow them to cook until the water has evaporated and beans tender
6. Add more water and cook for a little longer if needed
7. Season the beans with some salt and pepper
8. Enjoy!

Nutrition:

- Calories: 97
- Fat: 5.4g
- Carbohydrates: 7g
- Protein: 6.2g

Supremely Fascinating Lemon Chicken

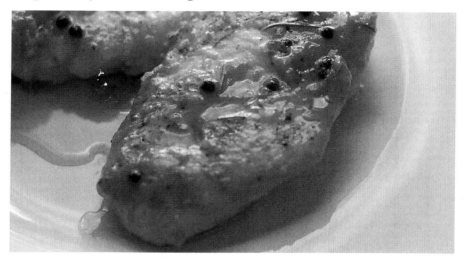

Prep Time: 10 minutes

Cooking Time: 15 minutes

Serving: 2

Ingredients:

- 2 skinless and boneless chicken breast halves cut up into 2-inch pieces
- ¼ piece of juiced lime
- ½ a juiced lemon
- 4 tablespoons of Dijon mustard
- Freshly ground black pepper
- Creole-style seasoning

Directions:

1. Take a skillet and place it over medium heat

2. Add chicken, lime and lime juices

3. Cook for a while and stir in black pepper, Creole seasoning, and Dijon

4. Mix well and keep cooking for 15 minutes until the chicken has reached doneness

5. Serve and enjoy!

Nutrition:

- Calories: 301
- Fat:3g
- Carbohydrates: 10g
- Protein: 55g

Feisty Crispy Fish Fillets

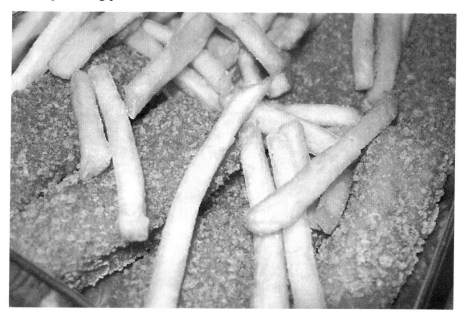

Prep Time: 10 minutes

Cooking Time: 10 minutes

Serving: 4

Ingredients:

- 1 whole egg
- 2 tablespoons of prepared yellow mustard
- 1/2 a teaspoon of salt
- 1 and a ½ cup of potato flakes
- ¼ cup of extra virgin olive oil
- 6 ounce of fish fillets

Directions:

1. Take a shallow sized dish and whisk in salt, eggs, and mustard
2. Keep the mixture on the side
3. Take another shallow dish and add potato flakes
4. Take a large sized heavy skillet and place it over medium-high heat
5. Add oil and allow it to heat up
6. Dip the fish into the egg mixture followed by the potato flakes
7. Fry in your hot oil for about 3-4 minutes per side until both sides are golden
8. Serve hot!

Nutrition:

- Calories: 391
- Fat: 18g
- Carbohydrates: 26g
- Protein: 30g

Mustard Drizzled Chicken

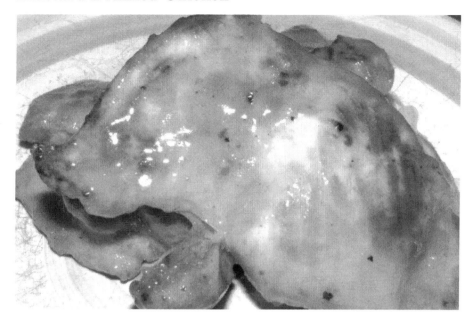

Prep Time: 15 minutes

Cooking Time: 60 minutes

Serving: 4

Ingredients:

- 4 pieces of skinless and boneless chicken breast
- 1 cup of prepared mustard
- 6 ounce of French Fried onions

Directions:

1. Pre-heat your oven to a temperature of 375 degrees Fahrenheit
2. Take a shallow dish and add mustard
3. Take another shallow dish and add onions
4. Dredge the chicken in mustard and coat them well
5. Dredge the chicken in the onion
6. Take a 9x13 inch baking dish and prepare it by greasing it up
7. Transfer the chicken to the baking dish

8. Bake for 50-60 minutes

9. Once done, take out and enjoy!

Nutrition:

- Calories: 442
- Fat:25g
- Carbohydrates: 21g
- Protein: 30g

Herbed up Cooked Chicken Breast

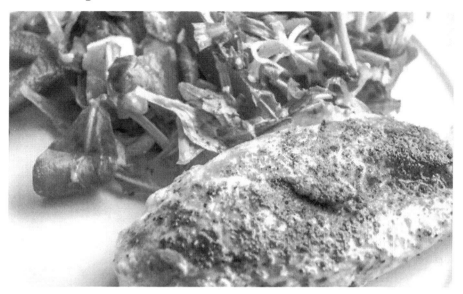

Prep Time: 10 minutes

Cooking Time: 20 minutes

Serving: 2

Ingredients:

- 3 tablespoons of extra virgin olive oil
- 1 tablespoon of minced onion
- 1 clove of crushed garlic
- 1 teaspoon of dried thyme
- ½ a teaspoon of crushed dried rosemary
- ¼ teaspoon of ground sage
- ¼ teaspoon of dried marjoram
- ½ a teaspoon of salt
- ½ teaspoon of ground black pepper
- 1/8 teaspoon of hot pepper sauce
- 4 bone-in chicken breast halves
- 1 and a ½ teaspoon of chopped up fresh parsley

Directions:

1. Pre-heat your oven to a temperature of 425 degrees Fahrenheit
2. Take a bowl and add olive oil, onion, garlic, sage, thyme, rosemary, hot pepper sauce, salt and pepper and mix everything well
3. This is your basting sauce
4. Turn the chicken breast into the sauce and coat it up well on all side
5. Take a shallow baking dish and add the marinated chicken breast, making sure to keep the skin side facing up
6. Roast in your oven for about 425 degree Fahrenheit for about 35-25 minutes, making sure to keep basting it from time to time using the drippings
7. Remove the breast to a warm platter
8. Spoon the pan juices over the breast and sprinkle some fresh parsley
9. Enjoy!

Nutrition:

- Calories: 391
- Fat: 21.9g
- Carbohydrates: 1.1g
- Protein: 45.1g

Sensual Portobello Mushrooms All Grilled up!

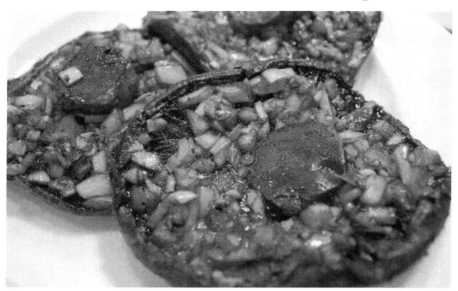

Prep Time: 10 minutes

Cooking Time: 10 minutes

Serving: 2

Ingredients:

- 3 Portobello mushrooms
- ¼ cup of extra virgin olive oil
- 3 tablespoons of chopped onion
- 4 minced clove of garlic
- 4 tablespoons of balsamic vinegar

Directions:

1. Carefully precious your mushrooms by cleaning them up and removing the stems
2. Keep the mushrooms for later use
3. Place the caps on a plate with the gills facing upward
4. Take a small sized bowl and add onion, vinegar, oil, and garlic

5. Mix everything well
6. Pour the mixture over the mushrooms caps and allow it to stand for about 60 minutes
7. Grill for about 10 minutes over your grill
8. Enjoy the grilled Portobello Mushrooms!

Nutrition:

- Calories: 217
- Fat: 19g
- Carbohydrates: 11g
- Protein: 3.2g

A Very Cool Lemon Pepper Chicken Dish

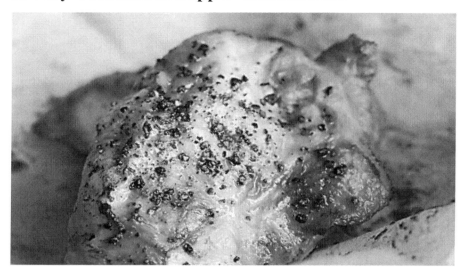

Prep Time: 10 minutes

Cooking Time: 30 minutes

Serving: 6

Ingredients:

- 6 skinless and boneless chicken breast halves
- 1 teaspoon of lemon pepper
- 1 pinch of garlic powder
- 1 teaspoon of onion powder

Directions:

1. Pre-heat your oven to a temperature of 350 degrees Fahrenheit
2. Take a 9x13 inch baking dish and grease it up nicely
3. Add the chicken to the dish
4. Season with garlic powder, onion powder, and lemon powder
5. Bake for 15 minutes
6. Turn the chicken over and add some more seasoning
7. Bake for another 15 minutes
8. Once the chicken is ready, serve and enjoy!

Nutrition:

- Calories: 133
- Fat:2.8g
- Carbohydrates: 0.5g
- Protein: 24g

Grandmother's Favorite Chicken Soup

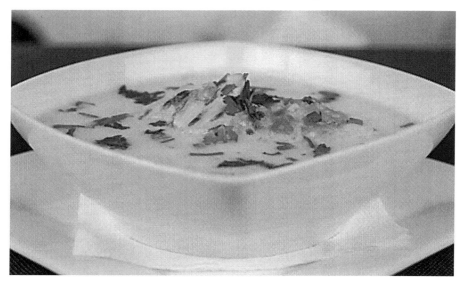

Prep Time: 10 minutes

Cooking Time: 15 minutes

Serving: 10

Ingredients:

- 1 piece of 3 pounds whole chicken
- 4 halved carrots
- 4 halved stalks of celery
- 1 halved large onion
- Water as needed
- Salt as needed
- Pepper as needed

Directions:

1. Take a large sized soup bowl and add chicken, carrots celery and onion

2. Cover and bring the water to a simmer

3. Keep simmer it until the chicken meat is tender and starts to fall off

4. Keep skimming off any excess foam

5. Take contents of the pot and strain the broth

6. Pick the meat off the bones

7. Chop up the carrots, celery, and onion

8. Add them to the broth

9. Season the broth pepper and salt

10. Return the pieced up chickens

11. Stir well

12. Serve!

Nutrition:

- Calories: 152
- Fat:9g
- Carbohydrates: 5g
- Protein: 13g

Sun Dried Artichokes Blessed With Tomatoes

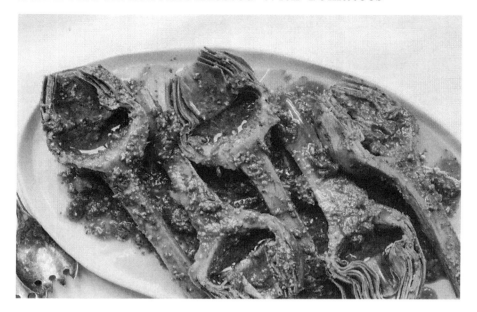

Prep Time: 10 minutes

Cooking Time: 25 minutes

Serving: 4

Ingredients:

- 4 boneless chicken breasts (skinless)
- Salt as needed
- Pepper as needed
- 2 teaspoons of extra virgin olive oil
- 14 ounce of diced tomatoes, green peppers, and onions
- ¼ cup of sun-dried tomato pesto
- 14 ounce of artichoke hearts (drained and quartered)

Directions:

1. Season both sides of the chicken breast with salt and pepper
2. Take a large sized skillet and place it over medium-high heat
3. Add oil and allow the oil to heat up

4. Add the chicken to the skillet and cook them, making sure that both sides are browned nicely
5. Remove the chicken from the skillet and place it on the side
6. Pour tomatoes into the pan and cook for 1 minute
7. Stir in artichokes, pest and lower down the heat to medium
8. Simmer the mixture for 10 minutes
9. Add the chickens to the pan and serve by giving it a nice stir!

Nutrition:

- Calories: 228
- Fat: 6.5g
- Carbohydrates: 11.4g
- Protein: 30g

The Constantly Evolving Shrimp Scampi

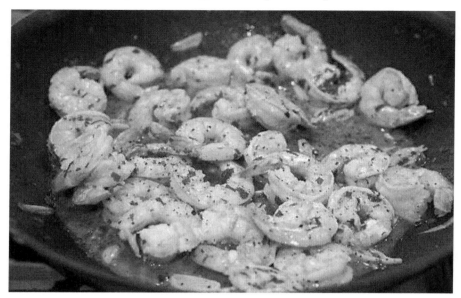

Prep Time: 30 minutes

Cooking Time: 6 minutes

Serving: 173

Ingredients:

- 4 tablespoons of ghee
- 1 tablespoon of extra virgin olive oil
- 4 minced garlic cloves
- ¼ teaspoon of red pepper flakes
- ¾ pound of shelled and deveined shrimp
- 1 tablespoon of lemon juice
- Zest of ½ a lemon
- 2 tablespoons of freshly minced parsley

Directions:

1. Pre-heat your oven to a temperature of 375 degrees Fahrenheit
2. Drizzle olive oil and season with salt and pepper

3. Place the cut side down on a baking sheet and bake for about 30 minutes

4. Take a large sized skillet and add ghee

5. Add olive oil and place it over medium-high heat

6. Add garlic and red pepper flakes and cook for 30 seconds

7. Add shrimp and cook for about 2-3 minutes per side until they are thoroughly cooked

8. Stir in parsley lemon juice and zest

9. Season with some salt

10. Enjoy!

Nutrition:

- Calories: 173
- Fat: 10g
- Carbohydrates: 1.6g
- Protein: 18.7g

Very Tangy Avocado and Cucumber Salad

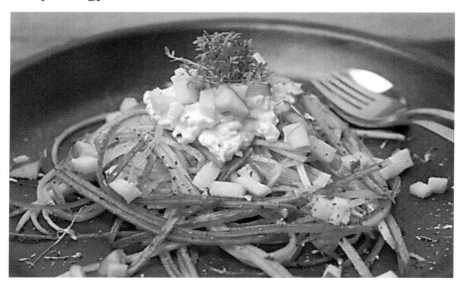

Prep Time: 15 minutes

Cooking Time: 0 minute

Serving: 4

Ingredients:

- 2 medium-sized cubed carrots
- 2 cubed avocados
- 4 tablespoons of chopped up fresh cilantro
- 1 minced garlic clove
- 2 tablespoons of minced green onions
- ¼ teaspoon of salt
- Black pepper as needed
- ¼ large sized lemon
- 1 piece of lime

Directions:

1. Take a large sized bowl and add cilantro, avocado and cucumber
2. Stir in pepper, onion, garlic and salt

3. Take lemon and squeeze on top
4. Toss everything well
5. Allow it to chill for 30 minutes
6. Serve and enjoy!

Nutrition:

- Calories: 186
- Fat: 14g
- Carbohydrates: 15g
- Protein: 3.1g

Obligatory Yellow Squash of Magic

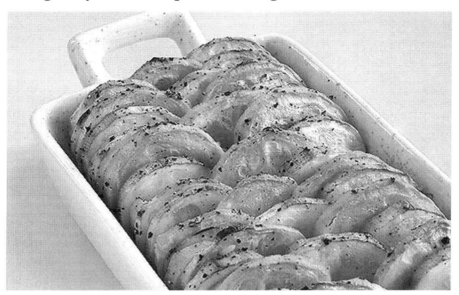

Prep Time: 10 minutes

Cooking Time: 10 minutes

Serving: 8

Ingredients:

- 4 medium-sized yellow squash
- ½ a cup of extra virgin olive oil
- 2 cloves of crushed garlic
- Salt as needed
- Pepper as needed

Directions:

1. Pre-heat your grill over medium heat
2. Cut up the squash horizontally and cut up into ¼ inch thick slices
3. Take a small sized pan and add olive oil
4. Heat it up
5. Add garlic cloves and cover it up

6. Cook over medium heat until the garlic starts to sizzle and a nice fragrant comes
7. Brush the slice of the squash with the garlic oil and season them with some salt and pepper
8. Grill the squash slices for about 10 minutes per sides until they reached the desired tenderness
9. Brush them up with some more garlic oil and enjoy!

Nutrition:

- Calories: 146
- Fat:14g
- Carbohydrates: 4g
- Protein: 1g

Juicy Coriander Pork Chops With Cumin

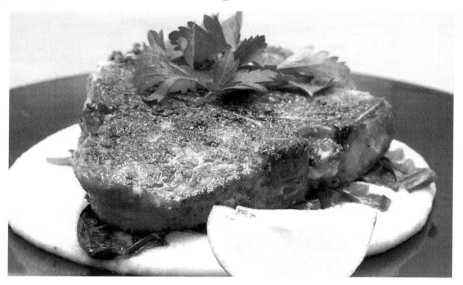

Prep Time: 10 minutes

Cooking Time: 15 minutes

Serving: 6

Ingredients:

- ½ a teaspoon of salt
- 1 tablespoon of ground cumin
- 1 tablespoon of ground coriander
- 3 minced garlic cloves
- 2 tablespoons of extra virgin olive oil
- 2 boneless pork loin chops
- Ground black pepper as needed

Directions:

1. Take a small sized bowl and add cumin, garlic, salt, coriander, 1 tablespoon of extra virgin olive oil and mix well to form a paste
2. Season the pork chops with some pepper and salt

3. Rub the chops with the paste
4. Take skillet and place it over medium heat
5. Add olive oil and heat it up
6. Add the chops and cook for about 5 minutes (per side) until the thickest part reads 145 degrees Fahrenheit

Nutrition:

- Calories: 278
- Fat:22g
- Carbohydrates: 5g
- Protein: 15g

Off the Ground Butternut Squash Fries

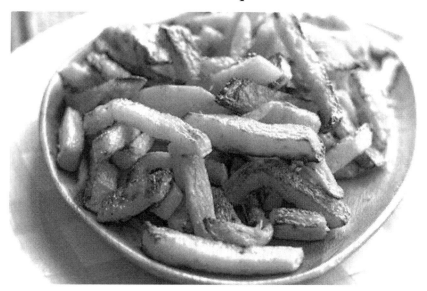

Prep Time: 15 minutes

Cooking Time: 20 minute

Serving: 4

Ingredients:

- 2 pounds of butternut squash (halved and seeded)
- Salt as needed

Directions:

1. Pre-heat your oven to a temperature of 425 degrees Fahrenheit
2. Take a sharp knife and peel the skin off
3. Cut up the squash into sticks resembling fries
4. Arrange the cut up squash into your baking sheet
5. Season them with some salt
6. Bake for 20 minutes making sure to give it a turn about halfway through
7. Once ready, serve crispy and hot!

Nutrition:

- Calories: 102
- Fat: 0.2g
- Carbohydrates: 26g
- Protein: 2.3g

Wall Street's Effective Carne Guisada

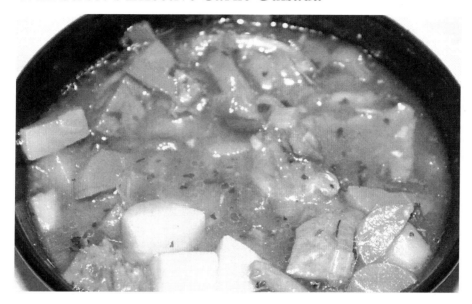

Prep Time: 15 minutes

Cooking Time: 120 minutes

Serving: 6

Ingredients:

- 8 ounce of tomato sauce
- ¼ cup of sofrito sauce
- .18 ounce of sazón seasoning
- 1 tablespoon of adobo seasoning
- ½ a teaspoon of dried oregano
- Salt as needed
- 2 pound of beef stew meat
- 2 cups of peeled and cubed potatoes
- 1 cup of water

Directions:

1. Take a large sized pot and add tomato sauce, sofrito sauce, sazón seasoning, salt, oregano, adobo seasoning and mix well
2. Simmer the mixture over medium-low heat for about 5 minutes
3. Add meat and cook until it is browned all over
4. Stir in water to cover the meat
5. Cover the pan and lower down the heat to low
6. Simmer for 60 minutes
7. Add potatoes and simmer for another 30 minutes until tender
8. Serve and enjoy!

Nutrition:

- Calories: 677
- Fat:46g
- Carbohydrates: 18g
- Protein: 44g

Hearty Lemon Ginger Shrimper

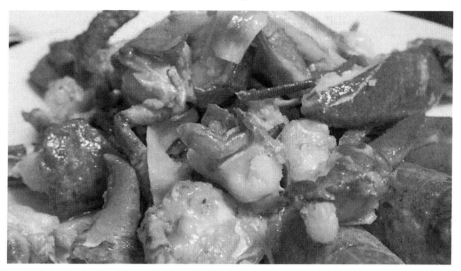

Prep Time: 20 minutes

Cooking Time: 6 minutes

Serving: 9

Ingredients:

- 3 pound of peeled and deveined jumbo shrimp
- ½ a cup of extra virgin olive oil
- ¼ cup of lemon juice
- 1 chopped onion
- 2 peeled cloves of garlic
- 2 tablespoons of grated fresh ginger root
- 2 tablespoons of minced cilantro leaves
- 1 teaspoon of paprika
- ½ a teaspoon of salt
- ½ teaspoon of ground black pepper
- Skewers

Directions:

1. Take a food processor and add olive oil, lemon juice, garlic, cilantro, onion, paprika, ginger, cilantro, pepper, salt
2. Blend well until a nice texture forms
3. Keep a little bit on the side for basting and pour the remaining mixture into a dish
4. Add shrimp to the dish and coat it well
5. Cover it and allow it to marinate for 2 hours
6. Pre-heat your grill over medium heat
7. Thread the shrimp onto skewers and discard any marinade
8. Lightly oil up the grate and grill the shrimp for 2-3 minutes, making sure to keep basting it
9. Use the leftover as sauce and enjoy!

Nutrition:

- Calories: 286
- Fat: 15g
- Carbohydrates: 4g
- Protein: 31g

The Genuine Southern Collard Greens

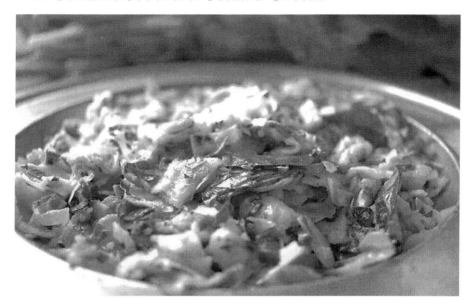

Prep Time: 15 minutes

Cooking Time: 60 minutes

Serving: 8

Ingredients:

- 1 bunch of rinsed and trimmed collard greens
- 2 smoked ham hocks
- 10 ounce of condensed chicken broth
- 21 fluid ounce of water
- 1 tablespoon of distilled white vinegar
- Salt as needed
- Pepper as needed

Directions:

1. Take a large sized pot and add collard greens and the ham hocks
2. Add chicken broth, water and vinegar
3. Season the mixture with some salt and pepper

4. Bring the whole mix to a boil and immediately lower down the heat once boiling point is reached
5. Allow it to simmer for 60 minutes
6. Serve and enjoy!

Nutrition:

- Calories: 165
- Fat: 11g
- Carbohydrates: 2.6g
- Protein: 12g

Perplexingly Satisfying Grilled up Lamb Chops

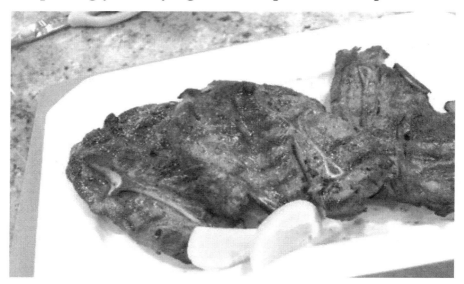

Prep Time: 10 minutes

Cooking Time: 6 minutes

Serving: 8

Ingredients:

- 4 cup of distilled white vinegar
- 2 teaspoons of salt
- ½ a teaspoon of black pepper
- 1 tablespoon of minced garlic
- 1 thinly sliced onion
- 2 pound of lamb chops

Directions:

1. Take a large sized re-sealable bag and add pepper, vinegar, salt, garlic, olive oil and onion
2. Mix well and wait until the salt has dissolved
3. Add lambs to the marinade and coat them well
4. Allow them to marinate for about 2 hours

168

5. Pre-heat your grill over medium-high heat

6. Remove the lamb from the marinade and discard it

7. Wrap up the exposed bones of your chop with aluminum foil

8. Grill for about 3 minutes if you are looking for a medium doneness

9. You may also broil the chops in your broiler (in case you don't have a grill) and broil for 5 minutes for a medium doneness as well

10. Serve and enjoy!

Nutrition:

- Calories: 519
- Fat: 44g
- Carbohydrates: 02.3g
- Protein: 25g

Savory Lebanese Chicken and Potatoes

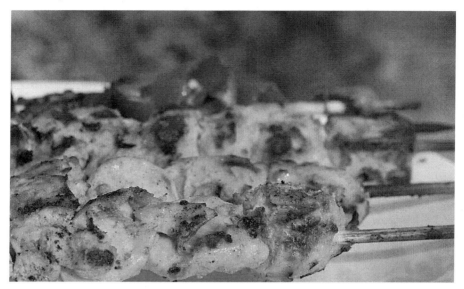

Prep Time: 15 minutes

Cooking Time: 60 minutes

Serving: 8

Ingredients:

- 8 cut up pieces of chicken
- 8 medium-sized potatoes (peeled and quartered)
- Salt as needed
- Ground white pepper as needed
- 4 cloves of crushed garlic
- 1 cup of fresh lemon juice

Directions:

1. Pre-heat your oven to a temperature of 425 degrees Fahrenheit
2. Take a large sized baking dish and add potatoes and chicken
3. Season them with some pepper and salt
4. Take a bowl and add olive oil, lemon juice, and garlic

5. Stir well and pour the mixture over chicken and potatoes (in the baking dish)
6. Cover the dish using a foil
7. Bake in your oven for about 30 minutes
8. Remove the foil (while still keeping the dish in the oven) and bake for another 30 minutes

Nutrition:

- Calories: 592
- Fat: 30g
- Carbohydrates: 53g
- Protein: 26g

Ever so Popular Lemon Eggplant

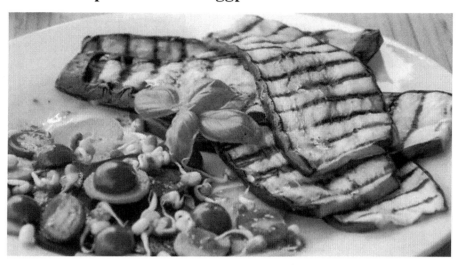

Prep Time: 15 minutes

Cooking Time: 25 minutes

Serving: 4

Ingredients:

- 1 large sized eggplant
- 3 tablespoons of extra virgin olive oil
- Salt as needed
- Pepper as needed
- 2 tablespoons of fresh lemon juice

Directions:

1. Pre-heat your oven to a temperature of 400 degrees Fahrenheit
2. Take a baking sheet and line it up with parchment paper
3. Slice up the eggplant into half-lengthwise and cut the halves into quarters
4. Cut up the halves into moons and add the prepared eggplants to your baking sheet
5. Make sure to keep the skin side facing down
6. Brush the eggplants with olive oil

7. Season with some pepper and salt
8. Roast the eggplants in the oven for 30 minutes until they are lightly browned
9. Remove and season with a bit of lemon juice
10. Serve and enjoy!

Nutrition:

- Calories: 120
- Fat: 10g
- Carbohydrates: 8g
- Protein: 1.2g

A Hard Bargaining Sesame Tilapia

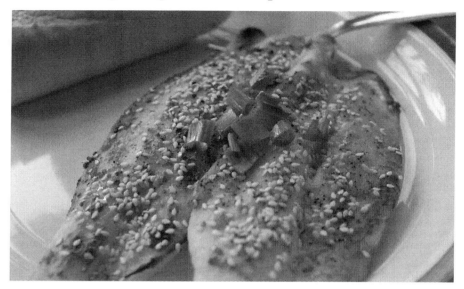

Prep Time: 15 minutes

Cooking Time: 30 minutes

Serving: 4

Ingredients:

- 2 pieces of 4-ounce fillets of tilapia
- ¼ cup of extra virgin olive oil
- 1 minced garlic clove
- 1 teaspoon of Italian seasoning
- Kosher salt as needed
- Fresh ground black pepper as needed

Directions:

1. Take a bowl and add the tilapia
2. Drizzle olive oil on top
3. Season the tilapia with Italian seasoning, kosher salt, pepper and garlic

4. Cover the tilapia up and allow it to marinate for about 30 minutes
5. Pre-heat your oven to a temperature of 350 degrees Fahrenheit
6. Transfer the Tilapia to a baking dish and bake for about 30 minutes
7. Once the fish is baked enough to be able to flake off easily, serve!

Nutrition:

- Calories: 359
- Fat: 28g
- Carbohydrates: 1.3g
- Protein: 23g

Oreganato Chicken Meal

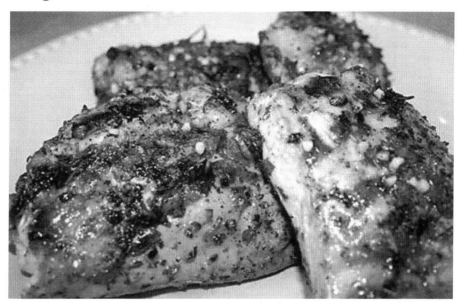

Prep Time: 10 minutes

Cooking Time: 40 minutes

Serving: 7

Ingredients:

- 7 pieces of chicken thighs
- 2 teaspoons of dried oregano
- Salt as needed
- ¼ cup of extra virgin olive oil
- ½ of a juiced lemon

Directions:

1. Pre-heat your oven to a temperature of 450 degrees Fahrenheit
2. Wash the chicken thoroughly and pat them dry
3. Take a small sized bowl and add salt and pepper to create a seasoning
4. Rub the chicken pieces with this prepared mixture

5. Take a 9x13 inch greased up baking dish and add the chicken

6. Take a bowl and whisk in lemon juice and oil

7. Drizzle half of the mixture over the chicken

8. Bake for about 15 minutes in your oven

9. Turn the chicken pieces over and drizzle the remaining mixture

10. Bake for 15 minutes

11. Enjoy!

Nutrition:

- Calories: 269
- Fat: 22g
- Carbohydrates: 1.1g
- Protein: 16g

A Homeless Man's Crazy Beef Meal

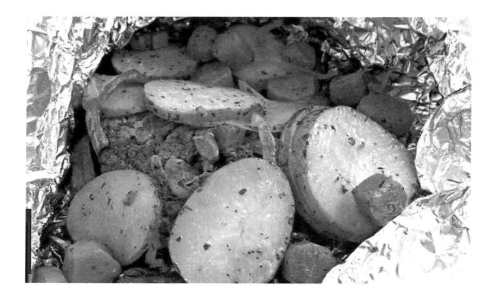

Prep Time: 15 minutes

Cooking Time: 60 minutes

Serving: 4

Ingredients:

- 1 pound of ground beef
- 5 peeled potatoes cut up into steak fries
- 4 large sized carrots peeled and sliced lengthwise
- 1 peeled onion sliced up into rings
- Salt vas needed
- Pepper as needed
- Garlic salt as needed

Directions:

1. Pre-heat your oven to a temperature of 400 degrees Fahrenheit
2. Take a 9x13 inch baking dish and line it up with aluminum foil

3. Shape up the ground beef into patties and place them in a nice layer in your pan

4. Layer up the vegetables on top of the beef patties, in the following order – potatoes, carrots, and finally onion rings

5. Season with some pepper, salt, and garlic

6. Cover with the foil

7. Seal up the edges

8. Bake for about 60 minutes

9. Enjoy once done!

Nutrition:

- Calories: 451
- Fat: 14g
- Carbohydrates: 56g
- Protein: 25g

Cute Salmon Cake

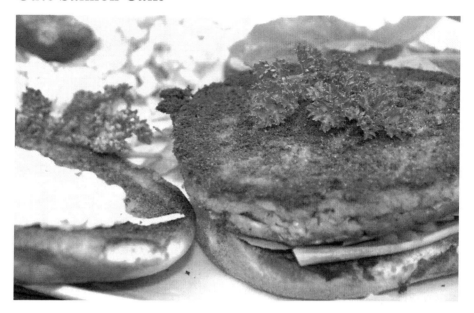

Prep Time: 10 minutes

Cooking Time: 20 minutes

Serving: 4

Ingredients:

- 14 ounce of drained and flaked salmon
- 2 beaten eggs
- 1 small sized diced onion
- 1 teaspoon of ground black pepper
- 3 tablespoons of extra virgin olive oil

Directions:

1. Prepare the salmon by picking the bones
2. Take a mixing bowl beat up the eggs
3. Add diced up onion, pepper, and salmon
4. Mix well
5. Add the salmon and mix everything well

6. Shape up 2-ounce patties
7. Take a large sized skillet and place it over medium heat
8. Add oil and allow it to heat up
9. Fry the patties for about 5 minutes (giving each side) until they have a golden brown texture
10. Enjoy once done!

Nutrition:

- Calories: 307
- Fat: 20g
- Carbohydrates: 2.3g
- Protein: 27g

Lemon Orange Tendersoft Roughy

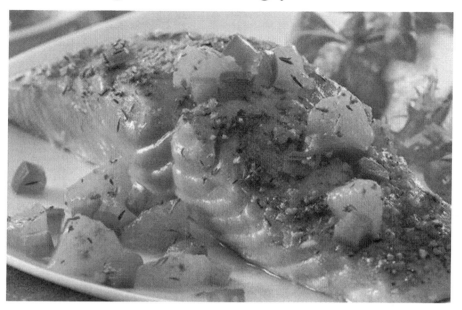

Prep Time: 15 minutes

Cooking Time: 5 minute

Serving: 4

Ingredients:

- 1 tablespoon of extra virgin olive oil
- 4 fillets of 4-ounce orange roughy
- 1 juiced orange
- 1 juiced lemon
- ½ a teaspoon of lemon pepper

Directions:

1. Take a large sized skillet and place it over medium-high heat
2. Add oil and allow it to heat up
3. Arrange the fillets in your skillets carefully
4. Drizzle orange juice and lemon juice on top
5. Sprinkle lemon pepper

6. Cook for about 5 minutes until the surface is flaky
7. Once fully cooked, enjoy!

Nutrition:

- Calories: 140
- Fat: 4g
- Carbohydrates: 8g
- Protein: 19g

Delicious Larger Than Life Steak

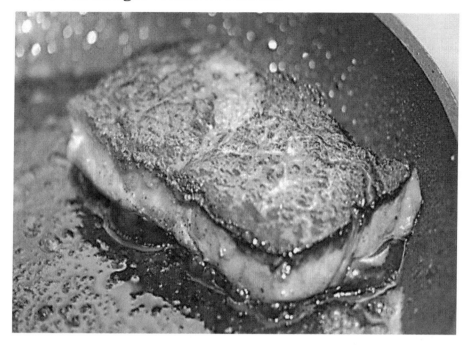

Prep Time: 15+10 minutes

Cooking Time: 60+180 minute

Serving: 4

Ingredients:

- 4 cube steaks

For French Onion Soup

- 5 pieces of onion cut up into ¼ inch half-moon slices
- 2 tablespoons of avocado oil
- 2-3 sprigs of fresh thyme
- Black pepper
- 5 cups of beef broth
- 1 tablespoon of tomato paste

Directions:

1. Take a large sized pan and add oil, thyme, and onion and place it over low heat

2. Cover with lid and allow it to steam for 20-30 minutes

3. Remove the pan lid and keep cooking for more 90 minutes

4. Make sure to stir it after every 30 minutes to avoid burning

5. Once the onions are deep, add tomato paste

6. Use just a splash of the stock to deglaze the pan and add the remaining stock

7. Simmer over low heat for about 60 minutes

8. The soup should be ready

9. Prepare by Pre-heating your oven to a temperature of 350 degrees Fahrenheit

10. Take a large sized skillet and place it over medium heat

11. Add cube steaks and cook them until they are nicely browned

12. Take a 13x9 inch baking dish and arrange the meat in a single layer

13. Pour soup on top and cover them up

14. Bake for about 60 minutes

15. Serve and have fun!

Nutrition:

- Calories: 435
- Fat: 22g
- Carbohydrates: 6.4g
- Protein: 49g

Tri-Top Juicy Grill With Oregano and Herbs

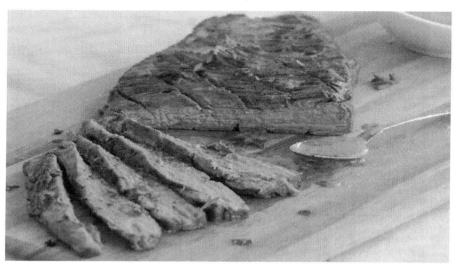

Prep Time: 15 minutes

Cooking Time: 1 hour15 minute

Serving: 10

Ingredients:

- 1 tablespoon of salt
- 1 and a ½ teaspoon of garlic salt
- ½ a teaspoon of celery salt
- ¼ teaspoon of ground black pepper
- ¼ teaspoon of onion powder
- ¼ teaspoon of paprika
- ¼ teaspoon of dried dill
- ¼ teaspoon of dried sage
- ¼ teaspoon of crushed dried rosemary
- 2 and a ½ pound of beef tri-tip roast

Directions:

1. Take a small sized bowl and add salt, garlic salt, celery, black pepper, onion powder, rosemary, dill and sage

2. Mix well and store it

3. Take a damp towel and carefully moisten the roast with water

4. Pat the roast with the prepared rub

5. Allow the meat to marinate for about 2 hours (or overnight). The longer you keep it, the deeper the flavors will seep in

6. Pre-heat your outdoor grill for high heat and oil the grate

7. Place the marinated roast on top and cook until all the sides are browned up

8. Remove it and reset your grill to medium-low (indirect heat) in case of a charcoal grill though, you can simply move the charcoal to the edge of the grill pit

9. Grill for 1 and a ½ hour for medium doneness

10. Remove and wrap with aluminum foil

11. Allow it to rest for 10 minutes

12. Carve it across grain slices and enjoy!

Nutrition:

- Calories: 214
- Fat: 9g
- Carbohydrates: 0.3g
- Protein: 30g

The Ancient Greek Roast of the Gods

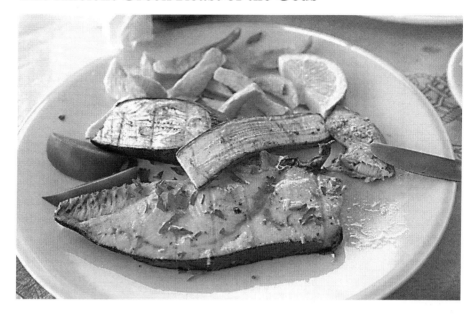

Prep Time: 10 minutes

Cooking Time: 50 minute

Serving: 2

Ingredients

- 5 small sized potatoes cut up into wedges
- 1 halved and sliced up onion
- 2 roughly chopped up garlic cloves
- ½ a teaspoon of dried oregano
- 2 tablespoons of extra virgin olive oil
- ½ of a lemon cut up into wedges
- 2 large sized tomatoes cut up into wedges
- 2 fresh skinless Pollock fish fillets
- Just a small handful of parsley

Directions

1. Pre-heat your oven to a temperature of 400 degrees Fahrenheit
2. Take a roasting pan and tip in onion, garlic, oregano olive oil
3. Season them well with mix everything well
4. Place the pan in your oven and roast for about 15 minutes
5. Add tomatoes and lemon
6. Roast for 10 minutes more
7. Top it up with the fish fillets and cook for another 10 minutes
8. Serve with Parsley scattered all around
9. Serve and enjoy!

Nutrition

- Calories: 388
- Fat: 13g
- Carbohydrates: 42g
- Protein: 23g

Chapter 11: Dinner Recipes

Subtly Caramelized Onion and Pork Chops

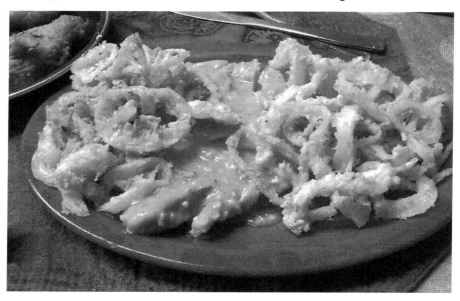

Prep Time: 5 minutes

Cooking Time: 40 minutes

Serving: 4

Ingredients:

- 1 tablespoon of extra virgin olive oil
- 4 ounce of pork loin chops of ½ inch thickness
- 3 teaspoons of seasoning salt
- 2 teaspoons of ground black pepper
- 1 onion cut up into strips
- 1 cup of water

Directions:

1. Take a small bowl and add 1 teaspoon of pepper and 2 teaspoons of seasoning salt
2. Take a skillet and place it over medium heat
3. Add oil and heat it up
4. Add pork chops and brown them on both sides
5. Add water and onions to the pan
6. Cover it up and simmer for 20 minutes
7. Turn the chops over and add more salt and pepper
8. Cover it up and keep cooking until the water evaporates and the onions are brown
9. Remove the chops and serve with onions on top!

Nutrition:

- Calories: 47
- Fat: 3.5g
- Carbohydrates: 4g
- Protein: 0.5g

Rich Guy's Lobster Tails

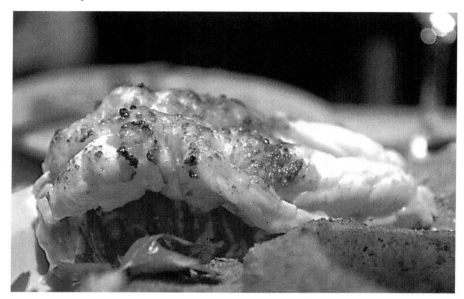

Prep Time: 15 minutes

Cooking Time: 12 minutes

Serving: 2

Ingredients:

- 1 tablespoon of lemon juice
- ½ a cup of extra virgin olive oil
- 1 teaspoon of salt
- 1 teaspoon of paprika
- 1/8 teaspoon of white pepper
- 1/8 teaspoon of garlic powder
- 10 ounce of rock lobster tails

Directions:

1. Set your grill to high heat
2. Take a small sized bowl and squeeze lemon juice
3. Whisk in olive oil and add paprika, garlic powder, salt and white pepper

4. Split the lobster tail lengthwise using a large size knife
5. Brush the fleshy side of the tail with marinade
6. Lightly oil up the grate of your grill and place the shrimp facing the flesh side facing downward
7. Grill for 12 minutes, making sure to give them a turn once! And keep bating them from time to time
8. Discard any excess marinade
9. Serve and enjoy!

Nutrition:

- Calories: 742
- Fat: 60g
- Carbohydrates: 4.3g
- Protein: 44g

The Old Folk's Aloo Phujia!

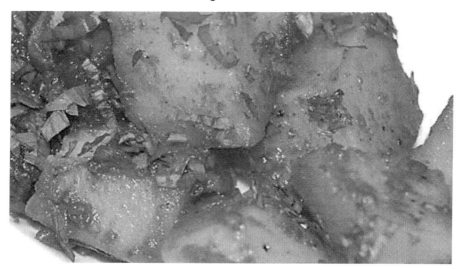

Prep Time: 10 minutes

Cooking Time: 20 minutes

Serving: 4

Ingredients:

- 1 chopped up onion
- ¼ cup of extra virgin olive oil
- 1 pound of cubed and peeled potatoes
- 1 teaspoon of salt
- ½ a teaspoon of cayenne pepper
- ½ teaspoon of cayenne pepper
- ½ teaspoon of ground turmeric
- ¼ teaspoon of ground cumin
- 2 chopped up tomatoes

Directions:

1. Take a medium-sized skillet and place it over medium heat
2. Add the oil and heat it up
3. Add onion to the oil and brown it

4. Stir in the turmeric, cayenne, salt
5. Add the potatoes and keep stirring it for 10 minutes
6. Add tomatoes and cover the pan for 10 minutes until the potatoes are tender
7. Serve!

Nutrition:

- Calories: 235
- Fat: 14g
- Carbohydrates: 25g
- Protein: 3.3g

Golden Rose Summer's Beach Party Special Shrimp

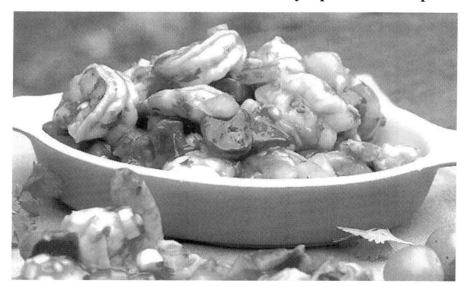

Prep Time: 10 minutes

Cooking Time: 10 minutes

Serving: 6

Ingredients:

- 1/3 cup of extra virgin olive oil
- 3 sliced garlic cloves
- 1 teaspoon of red pepper flakes
- 2 teaspoons of paprika
- 2 pound of deveined (shell-on) jumbo shrimp
- ¼ cup of lemon juice
- 2 tablespoons of chopped fresh basil
- ½ a teaspoon of salt
- ¼ teaspoon of black pepper

Directions:

1. Take a large sized skillet and place it over high heat
2. Pour oil and allow it to heat up

3. Add garlic and stir-fry well

4. Sprinkle a bit paprika and pepper flakes

5. Add shrimp and toss well to ensure that the shrimp has been coated up well

6. Pour lemon juice over the shrimp

7. Allow the shrimp to cook until a bright pink color is seen

8. Once done, cook for 1-2 minutes more

9. Lower down the heat to medium-low and add basil

10. Toss well

11. Season with salt and pepper

12. Enjoy!

Nutrition:

- Calories: 238
- Fat: 13g
- Carbohydrates: 2.2g
- Protein: 25g

Soft and Sweetly Created Minestrone Soup

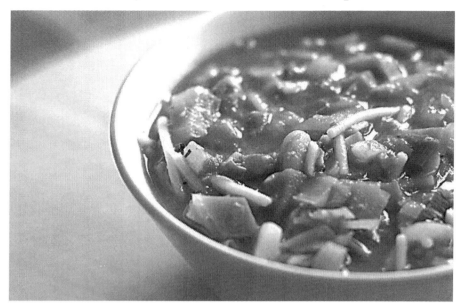

Prep Time: 30 minutes

Cooking Time: 5 minutes

Serving: 6

Ingredients:

- 1 tablespoon of extra virgin olive oil
- 1 chopped up large onion
- 2 chopped up large celery stalks
- 2 and a ½ teaspoon of Italian seasoning
- Salt as needed
- Pepper as needed
- 28 ounce of Italian Style Diced Tomatoes
- 5 cups of vegetable broth
- 2 large peeled and diced sweet potatoes
- 2 large thinly sliced carrots
- 6 ounce of green beans cut up into 1-inch pieces
- 5 minced garlic cloves

Directions:

1. Take a pot and place it over medium-high heat
2. Add oil and allow it to heat up
3. Add onion, Italian seasoning, salt, onion, pepper and Saute everything for about 5 minutes until tender
4. Stir in tomatoes, sweet potatoes, broth, carrots, garlic and green beans to the pot
5. Bring the mix to a boil
6. Lower down the heat to a simmer and allow it to simmer for 30 minutes, making sure to keep stirring it from time to time
7. Once the veggies are tender, serve and enjoy!

Nutrition:

- Calories: 201
- Fat: 2.7g
- Carbohydrates: 39g
- Protein: 4.5g

From The Sherlock Holmes Movies Goulash

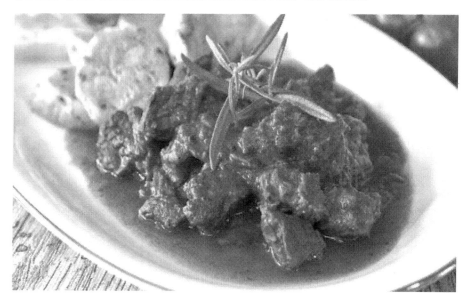

Prep Time: 15 minutes

Cooking Time: 120 minutes

Serving: 8

Ingredients:

- 3 tablespoons of lime juice
- 1 tablespoon of ground cumin
- 1 tablespoon of paprika
- 2 teaspoons of minced garlic
- 1 teaspoon of salt
- 1 teaspoon of black pepper
- 1 and a ½ pound of beef chunks
- 2 tablespoons of extra virgin olive oil
- 2 chopped onions
- 4 sliced large bell peppers
- 16 ounce of diced and drained tomatoes
- 16 ounce of coconut milk
- 1 bunch of chopped cilantro

Directions:

1. Take a large sized pot and place it over medium heat
2. Add oil and allow it to heat
3. Add onions and cook them until tender
4. Remove the onion and keep them on the side
5. Take a medium-sized bowl and add paprika, pepper, beef cubes and 2 teaspoons of salt
6. Mix well and add the cubes to the pot, cook until all sides are browned up
7. Return the onion to the pot
8. Add tomato paste, water, garlic and 1 teaspoon of salt
9. Lower down the heat to low and allow it to simmer for 2 hours until the meat is tender. Enjoy once done!

Nutrition:

- Calories: 549
- Fat: 42g
- Carbohydrates: 9.4g
- Protein: 32g

Healthy Bunch of Garlic, Onion, Cabbage and Rhyming Bacon!

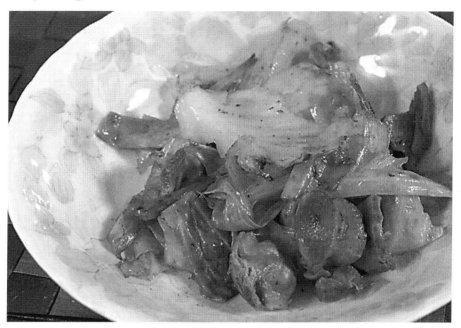

Prep Time: 15 minutes

Cooking Time: 60 minutes

Serving: 6

Ingredients:

- 6 large sized chopped bacon
- 1 diced large onion
- 2 minced garlic cloves
- 1 large cabbage head sliced and cored
- 1 tablespoon of salt
- 1 teaspoon of ground black pepper
- ½ a teaspoon of onion powder
- ½ a teaspoon of garlic powder
- 1/8 teaspoon of paprika

Directions:

1. Take a large sized stock pot and place it over medium-high heat
2. Add the bacon and cook for about 10 minutes until fully crispy
3. Add onion and garlic and cook for about 10 minutes more until the onions are caramelized
4. Stir in cabbage and keep cooking for 10 minutes
5. Season with some pepper, salt, garlic powder, paprika and onion powder
6. Lower down the heat to low and simmer for 30 minutes
7. Enjoy!

Nutrition:

- Calories: 194
- Fat: 12g
- Carbohydrates: 15g
- Protein: 6g

Fire and Ice Watermelon Salsa!

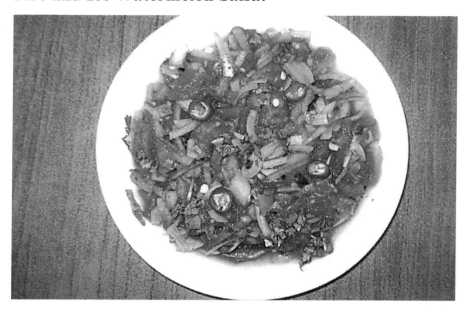

Prep Time: 15 minutes

Cooking Time: 15 minutes

Serving: 6

Ingredients:

- 3 cups of chopped up watermelon
- ½ a cup of chopped up green bell pepper
- 2 tablespoons of lime juice
- 2 tablespoons of chopped up fresh cilantro
- 1 tablespoon of chopped up jalapeno pepper
- ½ a teaspoon of garlic salt

Directions:

1. Take a small sized bowl and add watermelon, green bell pepper lime juice, cilantro, green onion, jalapeno, and garlic salt
2. Mix well

3. Serve the salad chilled!

Nutrition:

- Calories: 5
- Fat: 0g
- Carbohydrates: 1.3g

Exotic Kalua Pig!

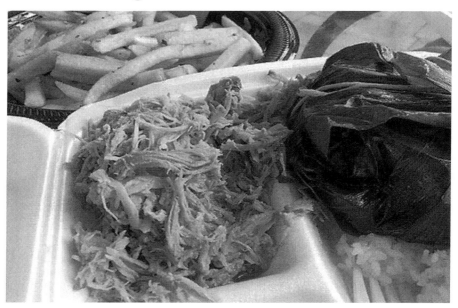

Prep Time: 10 minutes

Cooking Time: 20 hour

Serving: 12

Ingredients:

- 6 pound of pork butt roast
- 1 and a ½ tablespoon of Hawaiian sea salt
- 1 tablespoon of liquid smoke flavoring

Directions:

1. Take your pork and pierce it well all over using a fork
2. Rub salt all over and pour liquid smoke
3. Place the roast in your slow cooker
4. Allow it to cook for about 20 hours on low, making sure to give it a turn halfway through
5. Remove the pork
6. Shred the meat carefully and tear it apart

7. Enjoy with your favorite dipping!

Nutrition:

- Calories: 243
- Fat: 14.7g
- Carbohydrates: 0g
- Protein: 25.9g

The Best Trustworthy Brussels Sprouts

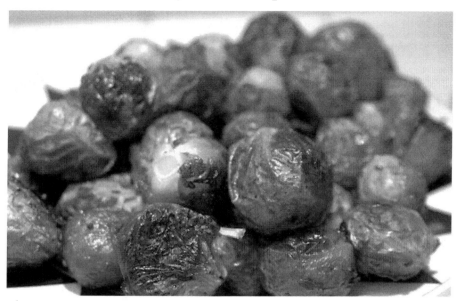

Prep Time: 15 minutes

Cooking Time: 45 minutes

Serving: 6

Ingredients:

- 1 and a ½ pound of Brussels sprouts with ends trimmed up
- 3 tablespoons of extra virgin olive oil
- 1 teaspoon of kosher salt
- ½ a teaspoon of finely ground black pepper

Directions:

1. Pre-heat your oven to 400 degrees Fahrenheit
2. Take re-sealable bag and add Brussels Sprouts, olive oil, kosher salt, and pepper
3. Shake the mixture well to allow the Brussels to get coated up well
4. Seal the bag tightly

5. Pour the Brussels into a baking sheet and place it in the center of your oven
6. Roast for about 45 minutes, making sure to give the tray a shake after every 5 minutes
7. Should you notice burning, you should lower down the heat
8. Once the sprouts obtain a brown texture, adjust seasoning and enjoy!

Nutrition:

- Calories: 104
- Fat: 7.3g
- Carbohydrates: 10g
- Protein: 2.9g

Generously Prepared Sugar Snapped Peas

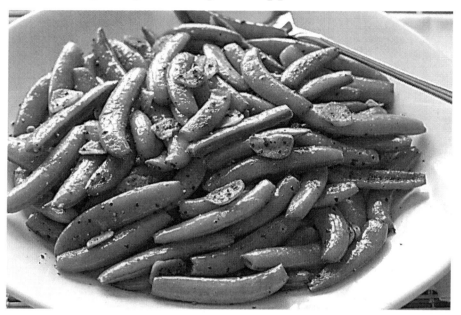

Prep Time: 10 minutes

Cooking Time: 8 minutes

Serving: 6

Ingredients:

- ½ a pound of sugar snap peas
- 1 tablespoon of extra virgin olive oil
- 1 tablespoon of chopped shallots
- 1 teaspoon of chopped up fresh thyme
- Kosher salt as needed

Directions:

1. Pre-heat your oven to 450 degrees Fahrenheit
2. Take a baking sheet and add sugar snap peas, making sure to form a single layer
3. Brush the peas with some olive oil
4. Sprinkle a bit of thyme, kosher salt, and shallots on top

5. Bake for about 6-8 minutes in your oven
6. Serve once they are tender!

Nutrition:

- Calories: 59
- Fat: 3.4g
- Carbohydrates: 5.3g
- Protein: 1.4g

Thinly Braised Balsamic Chicken Ala Gusto

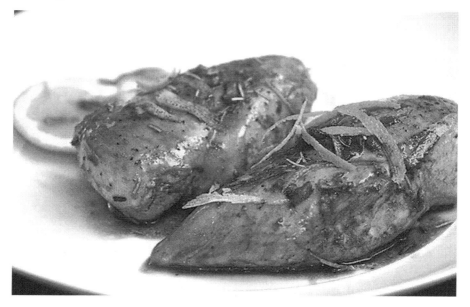

Prep Time: 10 minutes

Cooking Time: 25 minutes

Serving: 6

Ingredients:

- 6 boneless, skinless chicken breast halves
- 1 teaspoon of garlic salt
- Ground black pepper as needed
- 2 tablespoons of extra virgin olive oil
- 1 thinly sliced onion
- 1 can of diced tomatoes
- ½ a cup of balsamic vinegar
- 1 teaspoon of dried basil
- 1 teaspoon of dried oregano
- 1 teaspoon of dried rosemary
- ½ a teaspoon of dried thyme

Directions:

212

1. Season the chicken breast with garlic, salt, and pepper
2. Take a skillet and place it over medium heat
3. Add oil and heat it up
4. Add the chicken breast and cook for about 3-4 minutes each side until both sides are browned
5. Add onion and keep cooking for 3-4 minutes more
6. Pour the diced up tomatoes, balsamic vinegar over the chicken
7. Season with some oregano, thyme, rosemary, and basil
8. Simmer for about 15 minutes until the chicken is cooked well
9. The chicken is ready when it is no longer pink, and the internal temperature of the thickest part reads 165 degrees Fahrenheit. Enjoy once done!

Nutrition:

- Calories: 196
- Fat: 7g
- Carbohydrates: 7.6g
- Protein: 23.8g

Catchy Brazilian Fish Stew

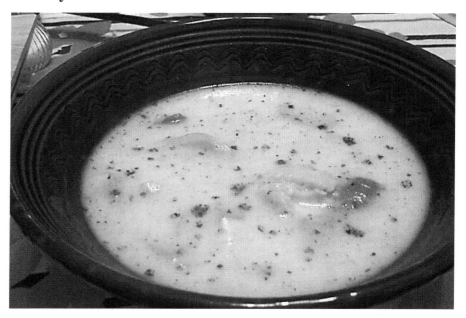

Prep Time: 20 minutes

Cooking Time: 25 minutes

Serving: 8

Ingredients:

- 3 tablespoons of lime juice
- 1 tablespoon of ground cumin
- 1 tablespoon of paprika
- 2 teaspoons of minced garlic
- 1 teaspoon of salt
- 1 teaspoon of black pepper
- 1 and a ½ pound of tilapia fillet cut up into chunks
- 2 tablespoons of extra virgin olive oil
- 2 chopped onions
- 4 sliced large bell peppers
- 16 ounce of diced and drained tomatoes
- 16 ounce of coconut milk

214

- 1 bunch of chopped off cilantro

Directions:

1. Take a bowl and add cumin, garlic, lime juice, pepper, paprika, and salt
2. Add tilapia and stir well to ensure that the fish is coated up
3. Cover the fish and allow it to chill for about 20 minutes (for quick cook) or 24 hours if you have the time
4. Take a large sized pot and place it over medium-high heat
5. Pour olive oil and allow it to heat up
6. Add onions to the oil and cook for 2 minutes
7. Lower down the heat to medium and add tilapia, bell peppers, diced up tomatoes
8. Cover and simmer for 15 minutes, making sure to keep stirring it
9. Stir in cilantro and cook for another 5-10 minutes. Serve hot!

Nutrition:

- Calories: 359
- Fat: 21g
- Carbohydrates: 15g
- Protein: 27g

Supergirl's Mother's Day Turkey Sausage

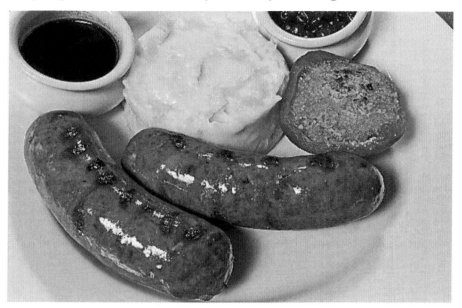

Prep Time: 5 minutes

Cooking Time: 15 minutes

Serving: 8

Ingredients:

- 2 pounds of ground turkey
- ¾ teaspoon of ground ginger
- 1 and a ½ teaspoon of salt
- 1 teaspoon dried sage
- ¼ teaspoon of cayenne pepper
- 1 and a ½ teaspoon of ground black pepper

Directions:

1. Take a large sized bowl and add ginger, ground turkey, salt and cayenne pepper
2. Mix and add sage and black pepper
3. Mix until blended well

4. Take a skillet and place over medium-high heat
5. Grease it up
6. Form sausages using the turkey mix and fry the patties for about 15 minutes until all sides are browned
7. Enjoy!

Nutrition:

- Calories: 169
- Fat: 8.6g
- Carbohydrates: 0.5g
- Protein: 22.5g

Basic Rattling Acapulco Chicken

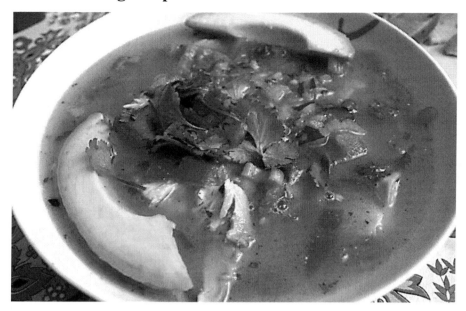

Prep Time: 10 minutes

Cooking Time: 15 minutes

Serving: 2

Ingredients:

- 2 skinless and boneless (halved) chicken breasts cut up into bite-sized pieces
- 1 tablespoon of divide chili powder
- Salt as needed
- Pepper as needed
- 1 tablespoon of extra virgin olive oil
- 1 cup of chopped up green bell pepper
- ½ a cup of chopped onion
- 2 jalapeno peppers minced and seeded
- 1 large sized tomato cut up into chunks
- 10 drops of hot pepper sauce

Directions:

1. Take your chicken and season it well with ½ a tablespoon of chili powder, salt, and pepper
2. Take a large sized skillet and place it over medium-high heat
3. Add oil and allow the oil to heat up
4. Add seasoned chicken and Saute for about 4 minutes
5. Remove the chicken from the skillet using a slotted spoon and keep it on the side, keep it warm
6. Add the onion and bell pepper to the very skillet and stir-fry
7. Add tomatoes, jalapenos, hot pepper sauce and ½ a tablespoon of chili powder
8. Cook for about 3-5 minutes, making sure to keep stirring them well
9. Return the chicken to skillet and fry for 2 minutes more
10. Enjoy!

Nutrition:

- Calories: 333
- Fat: 13g
- Carbohydrates: 23g
- Protein: 30g

Forever Together Courgette Salad

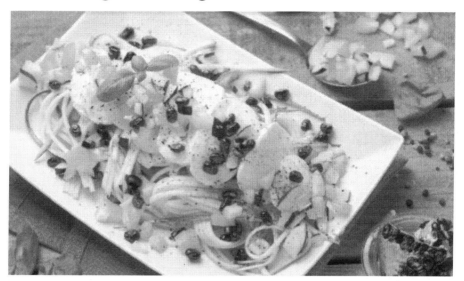

Prep Time: 20 minutes

Cooking Time: No cook required

Serving: 4

Ingredients

- 1 lemon juice
- 2 tablespoons of extra virgin olive oil
- ½ of a small pack of chopped up chives
- ½ of a small chopped up mint
- 300g of courgettes

Directions:

1. Take a large sized bowl and pour lemon juice
2. Season with some salt and pepper
3. Whisk in olive oil and add the chopped up herbs
4. Put Courgette through a Spiralizer using the noodle attachment
5. Tip the zoodles to your bowl

6. Add the prepped salad dressing to the bowl
7. Toss everything well
8. Serve and enjoy!

Nutrition

- Calories: 72
- Fat: 6g
- Carbohydrates: 2g
- Protein: 2g

Craziest Tom Ka Gai Ever!

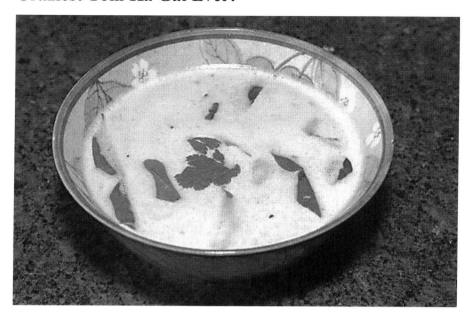

Prep Time: 30 minutes

Cooking Time: 5 minutes

Serving: 6

Ingredients:

- ¾ pound of skinless, boneless chicken meat
- 3 tablespoons of extra virgin olive oil
- 14 ounce of coconut milk
- 2 cups of water
- 2 tablespoons of minced fresh ginger root
- 4 tablespoons of fish sauce
- ¼ cup of lime juice
- ¼ teaspoon of cayenne pepper
- ½ a teaspoon of turmeric
- 2 tablespoons of thinly sliced green onion
- 1 tablespoon of freshly chopped cilantro

Directions:

1. Cut up the chicken into thin strips
2. Take a bowl and place it over medium heat
3. Add oil and heat it up
4. Saute the chicken strips for about 2-3 minutes
5. Take a pot and add coconut milk and water
6. Bring the whole mix to a boil
7. Lower down the heat to low and add fish sauce, lime juice, ginger, turmeric and cayenne powder
8. Simmer for 15 minutes
9. Sprinkle a bit of cilantro, scallion
10. Enjoy!

Nutrition:

- Calories: 433
- Fat: 41g
- Carbohydrates: 5.5g
- Protein: 14.8g

Steamed Cod Fish With Bizarre Lemon

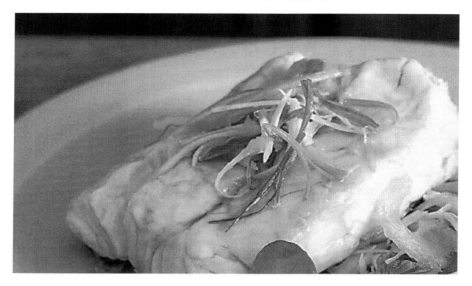

Prep Time: 25 minutes

Cooking Time: 40 minutes

Serving: 5

Ingredients:

- 6 ounce of halibut fillets
- 1 tablespoon of dried dill weed
- 1 tablespoon of onion powder
- 2 teaspoons of dried parsley
- ¼ teaspoon of paprika
- 1 pinch of salt
- 1 pinch of lemon pepper
- 1 pinch of garlic powder
- 2 tablespoons of lemon juice

Directions:

1. Pre-heat your oven to a temperature of 375 degrees Fahrenheit
2. Cut up a foil into 6 squares making sure that they resemble the size of your fillets
3. Center the fillets on the foil squares
4. Sprinkle dill weed, onion powder, parsley, paprika, lemon pepper
5. Season with salt and garlic powder
6. Sprinkle lemon juice on top of the fillets
7. Fold the foil over the fillet and make a pocket, fold from one edge to the other and seal it up
8. Place the sealed up packets on top of your baking sheet
9. Bake for 30 minutes until the fish flakes off
10. Serve and enjoy!

Nutrition:

- Calories: 142
- Fat: 1.1g
- Carbohydrates: 1.9g
- Protein: 29.7g

Spicy Harissa Infused Magnificent Chicken

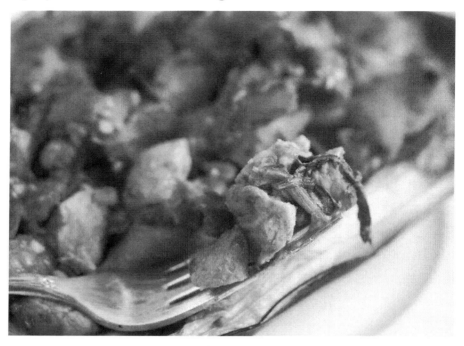

Prep Time: 10 minutes

Cooking Time: 30 minute

Serving: 4

Ingredients

- 1 large sized eggplant
- 2 tablespoons of extra virgin olive oil
- ¾ pound of organic chicken breast (Cubed up to small sizes)
- 1 chopped up onion
- 2 crushed garlic cloves
- 1 cup of chopped mushrooms
- 2 cups of fresh spinach
- 1 can of diced tomatoes
- 2 tablespoons of Mina Harissa Sauce

- 1 tablespoon of fresh basil
- 1 teaspoon of garlic granules
- Himalayan salt
- Red pepper flakes

Directions:

1. Pre-heat your oven to a temperature of 375 degrees Fahrenheit
2. Slice up the eggplant and scoop out the center of the eggplant
3. Keep it on the side
4. Brush up the eggplant with olive oil
5. Take a baking sheet and line it up with parchment paper
6. Add the eggplants and bake for about 15 minutes until they are tender
7. Take a skillet and place it over medium heat
8. Add 1 tablespoon of oil and heat it up
9. Add garlic and Saute them
10. Add the chopped up onion, chicken, mushrooms and chopped up eggplants
11. Keep cooking until the chicken shows an opaque texture
12. Add spices, tomatoes, and mina
13. Add spinach and mix well until everything is Sautéed
14. Add the mix to your scooped up eggplant and bake for 10 minutes
15. Serve and enjoy!

Nutrition

- Calories: 229
- Fat: 9g
- Carbohydrates: 7g
- Protein: 27g

Ultimate Tray Baked Fancy Fish

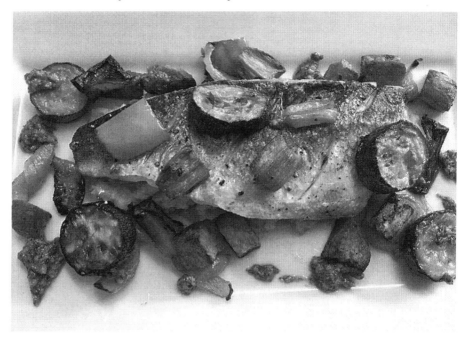

Prep Time: 10 minutes

Cooking Time: 30 minute

Serving: 2

Ingredients

- 300g of red skinned potatoes, sliced up into rounds
- 1 red pepper cut up into strips
- 2 teaspoons of extra virgin olive oil
- 1 sprig of rosemary with its leaves removed and finely chopped up
- 2 pieces of sea bass fillets
- 25g of pitted and halved black olives
- ½ of a thinly sliced lemon
- Just a handful of basil leaves

Directions:

1. Pre-heat your oven to 365 degrees Fahrenheit
2. Take a non-stick baking tray and arrange the potato slices
3. Add the pepper slices as well
4. Drizzle 1 teaspoon of oil on top
5. Season with some salt and pepper
6. Give everything a toss
7. Roast in your oven for about 12 minutes
8. Give the mixture a turn and bake for another 12 minutes
9. Arrange the fish fillets on top of the olives
10. Arrange the lemon slices on top
11. Drizzle a bit of more oil
12. Roast for 8 minutes more
13. Serve with some basil on top!

Nutrition

- Calories: 387
- Fat: 17g
- Carbohydrates: 28g
- Protein: 28g

Very Spicy but Mystically Sweet Green Chili Stew

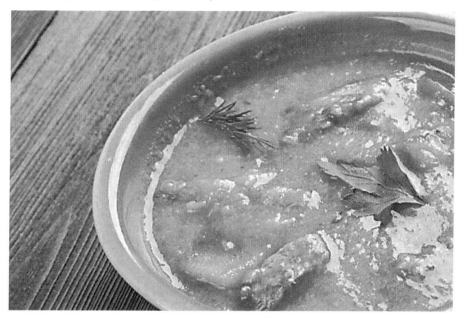

Prep Time: 15 minutes

Cooking Time: 90 minutes

Serving: 9

Ingredients:

- 1 tablespoon of extra virgin olive oil
- 2 pound of cubed beef stew
- 1 chopped onion
- 10 ounce of diced tomatoes with green Chile peppers
- 1 and a ½ cups of beef broth
- 4 ounce of chopped green Chile peppers
- 1 teaspoon of garlic salt
- 1 teaspoon of ground cumin
- Salt as needed
- Ground black pepper as needed
- 2 large sized peeled and cubed potatoes

Directions:

1. Take a large sized pot and place it over medium heat
2. Add oil and heat it up
3. Add the meat to the pot and brown for about 5 minutes (with onions)
4. Add diced in tomatoes, broth, Chiles and Chile peppers
5. Stir in garlic salt and cumin
6. Season with some pepper and salt
7. Bring the whole mix to a boil
8. Lower down the heat to low and allow it to simmer for about 60 minutes
9. Add cubed potatoes and simmer for another 30 minutes
10. Serve the soup hot!

Nutrition:

- Calories: 549
- Fat: 26g
- Carbohydrates: 33g
- Protein: 43g

Hasty Ethiopian Cabbage Meal

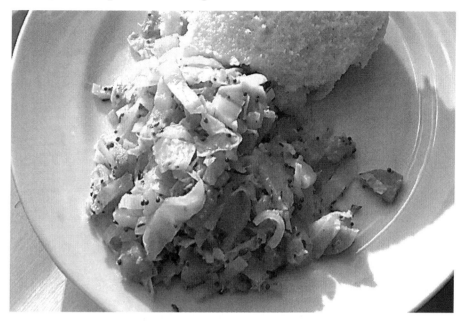

Prep Time: 25 minutes

Cooking Time: 40 minutes

Serving: 5

Ingredients:

- ½ a cup of extra virgin olive oil
- 4 thinly sliced carrots
- 1 thinly sliced onion
- 1 teaspoon of sea salt
- ½ a teaspoon of ground black pepper
- ½ teaspoon of ground cumin
- ¼ teaspoon of ground black pepper
- ½ teaspoon of ground cumin
- ¼ teaspoon of ground turmeric
- ½ of a shredded cabbage head
- 5 potatoes peeled and cut up into 1-inch cubes

Directions:

1. Take a skillet and place it over medium heat
2. Add oil and heat up
3. Add carrots and onion and Saute them for about 5 minutes
4. Stir in pepper, cumin, salt, turmeric, cabbage and cook for about 15-20 minutes
5. Add potatoes
6. Cover it up and lower down the heat to medium-low
7. Cook for 20-30 minutes until the potatoes are tender
8. Serve and enjoy!

Nutrition:

- Calories: 428
- Fat: 22.2g
- Carbohydrates: 54.1g
- Protein: 6.9g

A Darkened Broody Chicken

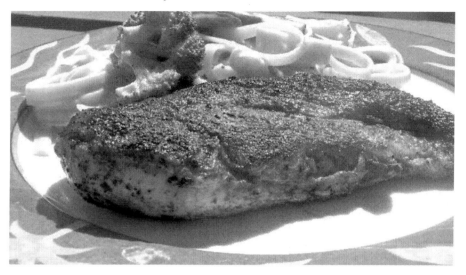

Prep Time: 10 minutes

Cooking Time: 10 minutes

Serving: 2

Ingredients:

- ½ a teaspoon of paprika
- 1/8 teaspoon of salt
- ¼ teaspoon of cayenne pepper
- ¼ teaspoon of ground cumin
- ¼ teaspoon of dried thyme
- 1/8 teaspoon of ground white pepper
- 1/8 teaspoon of onion powder
- 2 skinless and boneless chicken breast

Directions:

1. Pre-heat your oven to a temperature of 350 degrees Fahrenheit

2. Take a baking sheet and grease it up

3. Take a cast iron skillet and place it over high heat

4. Wait until it is smoking hot

5. Take a small sized bowl and add salt, cumin, paprika, cayenne, white pepper, onion powder and thyme

6. Take your chicken breast and oil it up with cooking spray on both sides

7. Rub the mixture all over the chicken breast

8. Place the chicken in your hot pan and cook for about 1 minute

9. Turn the chicken over and cook for another 1 minute

10. Transfer the baked chicken to the baking sheet and bake in your oven for 5 minutes

11. Serve and enjoy!

Nutrition:

- Calories: 135
- Fat: 3g
- Carbohydrates: 0.9g
- Protein: 24g

Zucchini Pasta for the Millennial

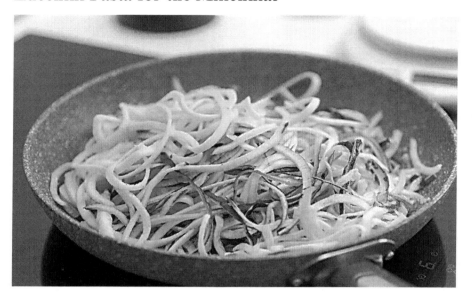

Prep Time: 10 minutes

Cooking Time: 5 minutes

Serving: 1

Ingredients:

- 2 pieces of peeled Zucchini
- 1 tablespoon of extra virgin olive oil
- ¼ cup of water
- Salt as needed
- Ground black pepper as needed

Directions:

1. Cut the zucchini lengthwise using a veggie peeler (make sure to stop once you have reached the seeds)
2. Turn the Zucchini and keep peeling until all sides have been peeled up into long noodle-like strips of zoodles
3. Discard the seeds
4. Slice up the pieces into spaghetti-like strips

5. Take a skillet and place it over medium heat

6. Add olive oil and heat it up

7. Add zucchini to the hot oil and fry for about 1 minute

8. Add water and cook for 5-7 minutes until the Zucchini are tender

9. Season with some pepper and salt

10. Enjoy!

Nutrition:

- Calories: 157
- Fat: 13g
- Carbohydrates: 8g
- Protein: 3g

Zinger Soft Calculative Tenderloins

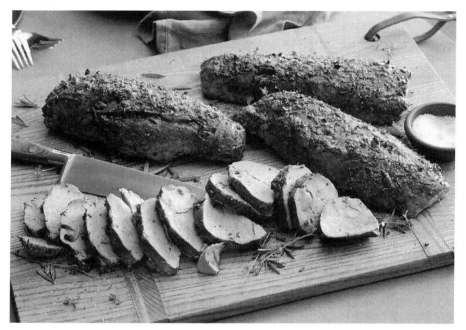

Prep Time: 15 minutes

Cooking Time: 30 minutes

Serving: 6

Ingredients:

- 1 and a ½ cup of fresh lime juice
- ¾ cup of extra virgin olive oil
- 6 sliced garlic cloves
- 2 teaspoons of salt
- 6 tablespoons of dried oregano
- 1 pound of pork tenderloins

Directions:

1. Take a large sized re-sealable bag and add lime juice, olive oil, garlic, salt and oregano
2. Shake the bag well to mix it up

3. Taste your marinade to check that the flavor is good
4. Add lemon for a more zingy flavor
5. Add tenderloins and allow them to marinate for about 2-5 hours
6. Pre-heat your grill over medium heat
7. Lightly oil up the grate
8. Discard the marinade and place the tenderloins to the grate and grill for 30 minutes
9. Enjoy!

Nutrition:

- Calories: 404
- Fat: 31g
- Carbohydrates: 9.1g
- Protein: 24g

A Simple Bowl of Spicy Cajun Shrimp

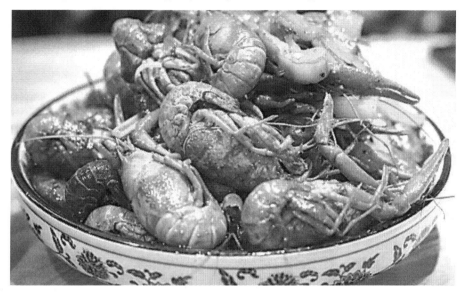

Prep Time: 5 minutes

Cooking Time: 15 minutes

Serving: 2

Ingredients

For the Dish

- 3 cloves of crushed garlic
- 3 tablespoons of ghee/clarified butter
- 20-30 pieces of jumbo shrimps

For the Cajun Seasoning

- 1 teaspoon of paprika
- Dash of cayenne pepper
- ½ a teaspoon of Himalayan Sea Salt
- Dash of red pepper flakes

- 1 teaspoon of garlic granules
- 1 teaspoon of onion powder

For Others

- 2 large pieces of spiraled zucchinis
- 1 sliced red pepper
- 1 sliced up onion
- 1 tablespoon of ghee/clarified butter

Directions:

1. Spiralize the zucchini using a Spiralizer
2. Take a bowl and add the ingredients listed under Cajun seasoning and add the shrimp
3. Toss the shrimp well
4. Take a pan and place it over medium heat
5. Add garlic and butter and allow it to heat up
6. Add onion and red pepper to the pan and Saute for 4 minutes
7. Add the seasoned Cajun shrimp to the pan and cook for a while until opaque
8. Take a separate heating pan and add a tablespoon of butter
9. Place it over medium heat and allow it to heat up
10. Add Zucchini and cook for 3 minutes
11. Add the cooked Zoodles to a bowl and top them up with the garlic Cajun shrimp and vegetable mix
12. Season with some salt
13. Enjoy!

Nutrition

- Calories: 92
- Fat: 7.6g
- Carbohydrates: 2.2g
- Protein: 4.6g

Super Zucchini Soup of Simplicity

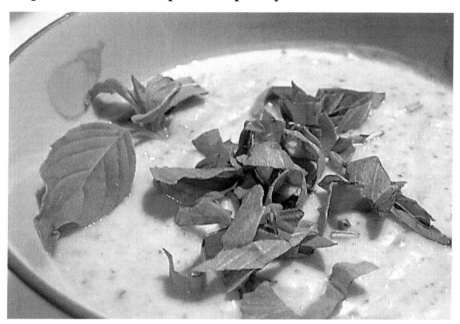

Prep Time: 25 minutes

Cooking Time: 60 minutes

Serving: 6

Ingredients:

- 2 tablespoons of extra virgin olive oil
- 1 large thinly sliced halved onion
- 1 tablespoon of curry powder
- Salt as needed
- 4 small sized zucchini halved up lengthwise and cut into 1-inch slices
- 1 quart of chicken stock

Directions:

1. Take a large sized pot and add oil
2. Place it over medium heat and allow the oil to heat up

3. Stir in onion and season them with salt and curry powder
4. Keep cooking until they are tender
5. Stir in zucchini and cook until they are tender
6. Pour chicken stock and bring the whole soup to a boil
7. Lower down the heat and allow it to simmer for about 20 minutes
8. Remove the soup
9. Use an immersion blender to blend the mix until smooth
10. Enjoy!

Nutrition:

- Calories: 74
- Fat: 5.2g
- Carbohydrates: 6.3g
- Protein: 1.8g

Amazing Spicy Pumpkin Chili!

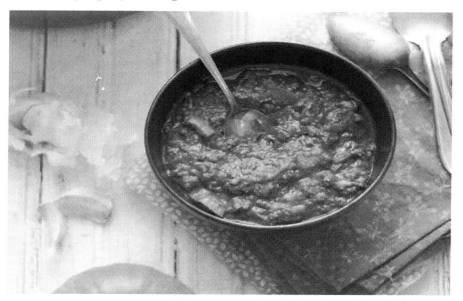

Prep Time: 10 minutes

Cooking Time: 15 minute

Serving: 2

Ingredients

- 3 cups of chopped up yellow onion
- 8 cloves of chopped up garlic
- 1 pound of ground turkey
- 2 can of 15-ounce fire roasted tomato
- 2 cups of pumpkin puree
- 1 cup of chicken broth
- 2 tablespoons of honey
- 4 teaspoons of chili spice
- 1 teaspoon of ground cinnamon
- 1 teaspoon of sea salt

Directions:

1. Take a large sized pot and place it over medium heat
2. Add coconut oil and heat it up
3. Add onion and garlic and Saute them
4. Add ground turkey and break it apart using a spatula
5. Cook for 5 minutes
6. Add the remaining ingredients and bring the whole mix to a simmer
7. Allow it to simmer for 15 minutes uncovered
8. Pour chicken broth
9. Serve with some salad!

Nutrition

- Calories: 312
- Fat: 16.2g
- Carbohydrates: 13.5g
- Protein: 27.4g

Travelers Hearty Rosemary Packed Chicken and Fries

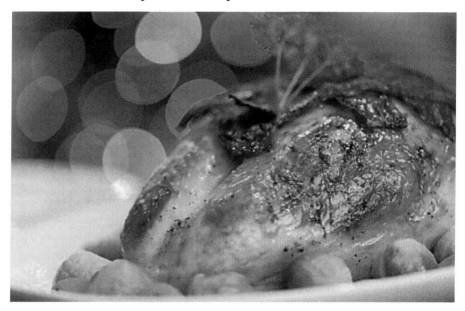

Prep Time: 15 minutes

Cooking Time: 60 minutes

Serving: 6

Ingredients:

- 8 pieces of chicken thigh
- 6 small quartered red potatoes
- ½ a cup of extra virgin olive oil
- 1 tablespoon of chopped up fresh rosemary
- 1 and a ½ teaspoon of chopped up fresh oregano
- 1 and a ½ teaspoon of garlic powder
- Salt as needed
- Pepper as needed

Directions:

1. Pre-heat your oven to a temperature of 375 degrees Fahrenheit
2. Take a large sized bowl and add potatoes and chicken
3. Pour olive oil and stir everything to ensure that the chicken has been coated up
4. Take a large sized baking dish and scatter the potato pieces and chicken on it
5. Sprinkle oregano, garlic powder, rosemary, pepper and salt
6. Bake for 60 minutes making sure to keep basting it during the final 15 minutes
7. Enjoy!

Nutrition:

- Calories: 497
- Fat: 31g
- Carbohydrates: 27g
- Protein: 24.4g

Planetary Roast of Vegetables

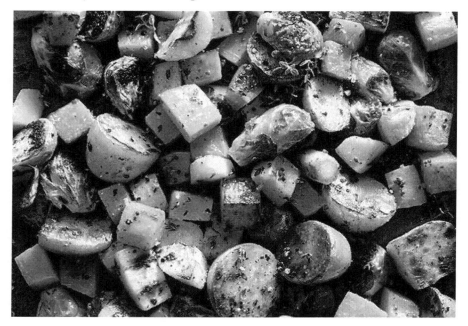

Prep Time: 25 minutes

Cooking Time: 60 minutes

Serving: 6

Ingredients:

- 2 tablespoons of extra virgin olive oil
- 1 large peeled yam cut up into 1-inch pieces
- 1 large parsnips peeled and cut up into 1-inch pieces
- 1 cup of baby carrots
- 1 zucchini cut up into 1-inch slices
- 1 bunch of fresh asparagus, trimmed up into 1-inch pieces
- ½ a cup of roasted red peppers cut up into 1-inch pieces
- 2 minced garlic cloves
- ¼ cup of chopped up fresh basil
- ½ a teaspoon of kosher salt
- ½ a teaspoon of ground black pepper

Directions:

1. Pre-heat your oven to a temperature of 425 degrees Fahrenheit
2. Take 2 baking sheets and grease them up 1 tablespoon of olive oil
3. Add parsnips, carrots, and yam
4. Bake for 30 minutes
5. Add asparagus, zucchini and 1 tablespoon of olive oil
6. Bake for another 30 minutes until the veggies are tender
7. Once done, remove and allow the oven to cool
8. Add roasted peppers alongside basil, pepper, garlic, salt in a large sized bowl
9. Add the roasted vegetable to the bowl and give the mixture a toss. Serve chilled and enjoy!

Nutrition:

- Calories: 191
- Fat: 5g
- Carbohydrates: 34g
- Protein: 4g

Original African Chicken Dish

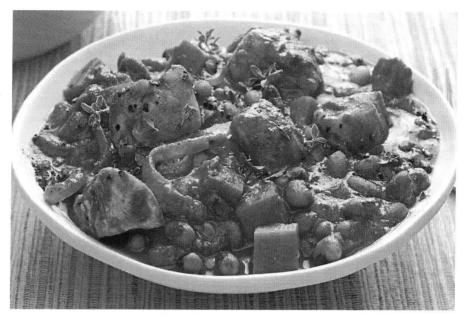

Prep Time: 20 minutes

Cooking Time: 40 minute

Serving: 4

Ingredients

- 1 tablespoon of extra virgin olive oil
- 1 chopped up onion
- 2 cloves of peeled garlic
- 1 piece of bay leaf
- 14.5 ounce of whole peeled tomatoes
- 2 teaspoons of curry powder
- 1/8 teaspoon of salt
- 2-3 pound of whole chicken with the bones and skin, and the chicken cut up into pieces
- 1 juice lemon

Directions:

1. Take a heavy skillet and place it over medium heat
2. Add oil and allow it to heat up
3. Stir in garlic, bay leaf, and onion and Saute until the onions are nicely browned up
4. Add curry powder, salt and tomatoes, and salt
5. Cook for about 5 minutes
6. Add the chicken now and cook for about 20 minutes
7. Lower down the heat to low and simmer for 10 minutes, while gradually adding the coconut milk slowly
8. Add lemon juice and enjoy!

Nutrition

- Calories: 600
- Fat: 33g
- Carbohydrates: 13g
- Protein: 64g

Childish Mangetout and Papaya Medley

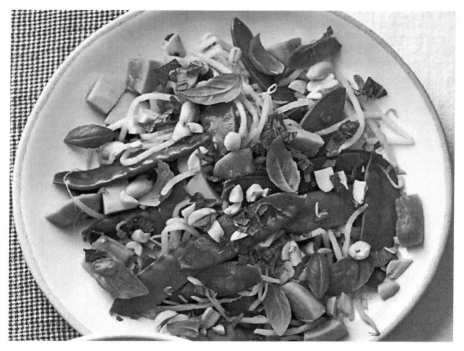

Prep Time: 10 minutes

Cooking Time: 5 minute

Serving: 2

Ingredients

- 175g of Mangetout
- 175g of beansprouts
- 1 peeled and deseeded papaya cut up into cubes
- 1 juice of the lime
- A small handful of torn basil leaves
- Small handful of chopped up mint leaves

Directions:

1. Take a large sized skillet and place it over high heat
2. Add Mangetout and 1 tablespoon of water
3. Cook for a while
4. Add beansprouts and cook for about 2-3 minutes
5. Remove the heat
6. Add papaya and lime juice
7. Add herbs
8. Give it a toss
9. And enjoy!

Nutrition

- Calories: 198
- Fat: 7g
- Carbohydrates: 21g
- Protein: 10g

Lime and Chicken Authentic Indian Kabob!

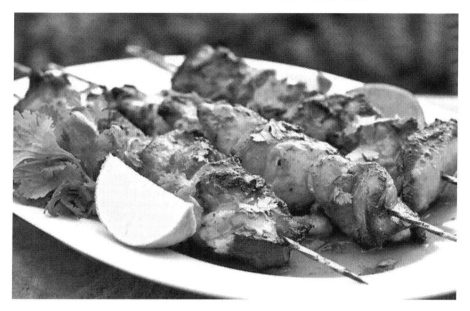

Prep Time: 15 minutes

Cooking Time: 15 minutes

Serving: 4

Ingredients:

- 3 tablespoons of extra virgin olive oil
- 1 and a ½ tablespoon of red wine vinegar
- 1 juiced lime
- 1 teaspoon of chili powder
- ½ a teaspoon of paprika
- ½ a teaspoon of onion powder
- ½ a teaspoon of garlic powder
- Cayenne pepper
- Salt as needed
- Freshly ground pepper as needed
- 1 pound of skinless, boneless halved chicken breast
- Skewers

Directions:

1. Take a small sized bowl and whisk in vinegar, olive oil, lime juice
2. Season with some chili powder, paprika, onion powder, garlic powder, cayenne pepper, salt and black pepper
3. Add chicken to a shallow baking dish and pour the prepared sauce
4. Stir well to coat things up
5. Cover and allow it to chill for 60 minutes
6. Pre-heat your grill over high heat
7. Thread the chicken onto skewers and discard the marinade
8. Lightly oil up your grate and grill for 10-15 minutes
9. Enjoy!

Nutrition:

- Calories: 227
- Fat: 13g
- Carbohydrates: 3.2g
- Protein: 23.9

Conclusion

I would like to thank you for purchasing this book and as well as taking your time to read through.

I do hope that this book has been helpful and you found the information useful!

Keep in mind that you are not only limited to the recipes provided in this book! Just go ahead and keep on exploring until you find the perfect recipes for your next life-changing 30 days!

Stay healthy and stay safe!

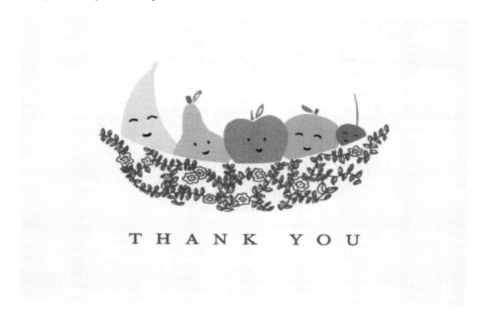

T H A N K   Y O U

Made in the USA
San Bernardino, CA
24 January 2018